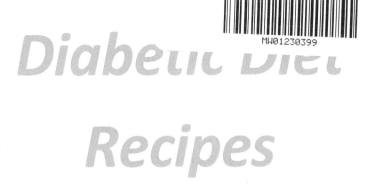

Diabetic Diet

Recipes

Tasty Low-Carb Recipes for Diabetic and Pre-Diabetic People

Rose Hill

render any resulting actions solely under their purview. There are no scenarios in which the publisher or the original author of this work can be in any fashion deemed liable for any hardship or damages that may befall them after undertaking information described herein.

Additionally, the information in the following pages is intended only for informational purposes and should thus be thought of as universal. As befitting its nature, it is presented without assurance regarding its prolonged validity or interim quality. Trademarks that are mentioned are done without written consent and can in no way be considered an endorsement from the trademark holder.

Table of Contents

Introduction

Diabetes is not only treated with anti-diabetic drugs or insulin but necessarily with:

Diet - If you think that avoiding sugar or replacing refined carbohydrates with whole-grain ones is correct, unfortunately, it is not. You'll have to learn how to introduce carbohydrates, without exceeding the daily doses, associating proteins and fats with the meals.

Lifestyle - If you are overweight you will have to lose weight by reducing the percentage of carbohydrates. If you are very stressed, nervous, you should dedicate yourself to relaxing activities: recent studies have shown how yoga, mindfulness, improve diabetes.

Regular physical activity - It is advisable to have a minimum daily physical activity of 30 minutes per day to be able to reach 60 minutes. Physical activity should be moderate-intensity such as walking, biking, swimming, dancing. The activity should be a mix of cardiovascular, stretching, and resistance activities to maintain or increase lean body mass. Physical activity increases glucose consumption by muscles, reduces insulin resistance, loses weight more easily while feeling better.

Following a controlled and healthy diet serves above all to keep the blood sugar level under control, through a correct dietary intake of all the nutrients necessary for the health of the body.

If it is not necessary to lose weight quickly, the ideal diet for diabetes is not at all complex or restrictive.

A person with diabetes needs a daily caloric intake equal to that of the non-diabetic subject, to factors such as physical constitution, sex, age, height, and work activity, having as objective the achievement and maintenance of the ideal body weight.

In the daily diet, must be carefully evaluated the intake of simple sugars with rapid absorption (glucose and sucrose) giving preference to complex sugars with slow absorption (starch).

The total daily intake of carbohydrates should not exceed 50-55% of total calories, provided that at least 80% of it is starch and the remaining 20% is non-insulin-dependent sugars and fiber.

Fibers must be taken in high quantities, especially the water-soluble ones, capable of slowing down the intestinal absorption of carbohydrates and cholesterol.

Proteins must make up about 15%-20% of total calories and at least one-third must be animal proteins, rich in essential amino acids.

The remaining calories (25%-30%) must be provided by fats, possibly of vegetable origin, with a high content of polyunsaturated fatty acids, useful in the prevention of cardiovascular diseases. The intake of vitamins and mineral salts must also be adequate. In this book, the author collects some of the tastiest and easiest recipes for every day.

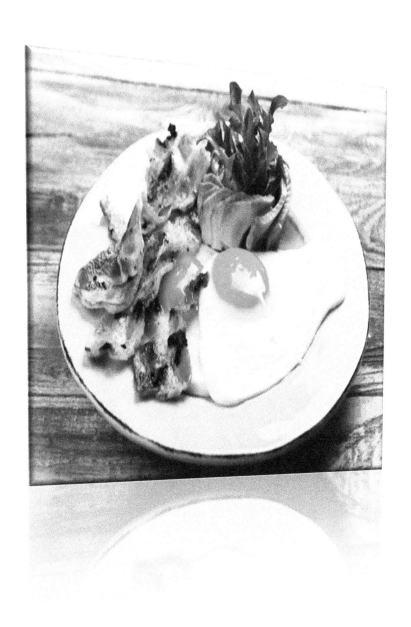

Breakfast Recipes

Slow "Roasted" Tomatoes

TIME TO PREPARE
5 minutes

COOK TIME
1hour 15 minutes

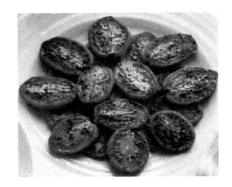

SERVING
2 People

Ingredients

- ½ tablespoon balsamic vinegar
- 1 large firm under-ripe tomato, halved crosswise
- 1 garlic clove, minced
- 1 teaspoon olive oil
- ½ teaspoon dried basil, crushed
- ½ cup breadcrumbs, coarse, soft whole-wheat
- Dried rosemary, crushed
- 1 tablespoon Parmesan cheese, grated
- Salt
- ¼ teaspoon dried oregano, crushed

Steps to Cook

1. Using cooking spray, coat the unheated slow cooker lightly. Then add tomatoes to the bottom of the slow cooker, cut side up.
2. In a bowl, combine vinegar together with garlic, oil, rosemary, dried basil, and salt, and then spoon the mixture over the tomatoes in the slow cooker evenly.
3. Close the lid and cook for either 2 hours on low, or 1 hour on high.
4. Over medium heat, preheat a skillet, and then add the breadcrumbs. Cook as you stir constantly until lightly browned, for about 2-3 minutes. Remove from heat when done and then stir in the parmesan.

- *Chopped fresh basil, optional*

5. When through, remove tomatoes from the slow cooker and put them on the serving plates, and then drizzle over tomatoes with the cooking liquid. Then sprinkle with the breadcrumb mixture and let rest for 10 minutes in order to absorb the flavors.
6. Garnish with basil if need be and then serve. Enjoy!

Rhubarb Muffins

TIME TO PREPARE
10 minutes

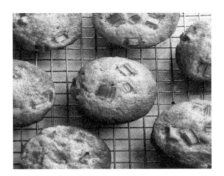

SERVING
8 People

COOK TIME
25 minutes

Ingredients

- ½ cup almond meal
- 2 tablespoons crystallized ginger
- ¼ cup coconut sugar
- 1 tablespoon linseed meal
- ½ cup buckwheat flour
- ¼ cup brown rice flour
- 2 tablespoons powdered arrowroot
- 2 teaspoon gluten-free baking powder
- ½ teaspoon fresh grated ginger
- ½ teaspoon ground cinnamon

Steps to Cook

1. In a bowl, mix the almond meal with the crystallized ginger, sugar, linseed meal, buckwheat flour, rice flour, arrowroot powder, grated ginger, baking powder, and cinnamon, and stir. In another bowl, mix the rhubarb with the apple, almond milk, oil, egg, and vanilla and stir well. Combine the 2 mixtures, stir well, and divide into a lined muffin tray. Place in the oven at 350 degrees F and bake for 25 minutes. Serve the muffins for breakfast.

2. Enjoy!

- *1 cup rhubarb, sliced*
- *1 apple, cored, peeled, and chopped*
- *1/3 cup almond milk, unsweetened*
- *¼ cup olive oil 1 free-range egg*
- *1 teaspoon vanilla extract*

Fried Egg with Bacon

TIME TO PREPARE
5 minutes

COOK TIME
10 minutes

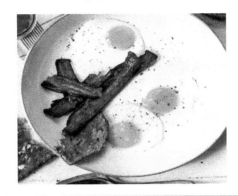

SERVING
1 People

Ingredients

- *2 eggs*
- *30 grams of bacon*
- *2 tablespoon olive oil*
- *salt & pepper*

Steps to Cook

1. Heat oil in the pan and fry the bacon.
2. Reduce the heat and beat the eggs in the pan.
3. Cook the eggs and season with salt and pepper.
4. Serve the fried eggs hot with the bacon.

Almond Flour Porridge

TIME TO PREPARE
5 minutes

COOK TIME
5 minutes

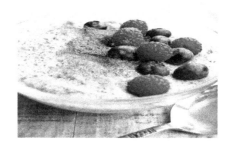

SERVING
1 People

Ingredients

- 1 tsp. Erythritol, granulated
- 2 tbsp. Flaxseed, grounded
- ½ cup Almond Milk, unsweetened
- 2 tbsp. Almond Flour
- 2 tbsp. Sesame Seeds, grounded

Steps to Cook

1. Combine the sesame seeds, flaxseed meal, and almond flour in a microwave-safe bowl and mix well.
2. To this, pour the almond milk and heat it on high power for one minute in the microwave.
3. Stir in the mixture and heat it again for one minute. Add more milk if the mixture seems thicker.
4. Sprinkle the erythritol over it and combine it. Tip: You can top it with berries if desired.

Coconut Pancakes

TIME TO PREPARE
5 minutes

COOK TIME
15 minutes

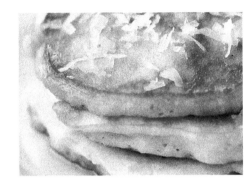

SERVING
4 People

Ingredients

- 1 cup coconut flour
- 2 tablespoons of arrowroot powder
- 1 teaspoon. baking powder
- 1 cup of coconut milk
- 3 tablespoons coconut oil

Steps to Cook

1. In a medium container, mix the dry ingredients all together.
2. Add the coconut milk and a couple of tablespoons of the copra oil, then mix properly.
3. In a skillet, melt 1 teaspoon of copra oil.
4. Pour a ladle of the batter into the skillet, then swirl the pan to spread the batter evenly into a smooth pancake.
5. Cook it for like 3 minutes on medium heat until it becomes firm.
6. Turn the pancake to the other side, then cook it for an additional 2 minutes until it turns golden brown.
7. Cook the remaining pancakes in the same process.
8. Serve.

Baked Mini Quiche

TIME TO PREPARE
10 minutes

COOK TIME
15 minutes

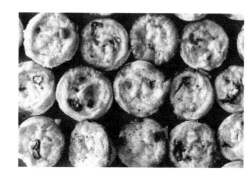

SERVING
2 People

Ingredients

- *2 eggs*
- *1 large yellow onion, diced*
- *1 ¾ cups whole wheat flour*
- *1 ½ cups spinach, chopped*
- *¾ cup cottage cheese*
- *Salt and black pepper to taste*
- *2 tablespoons olive oil*
- *¾ cup butter*
- *¼ cup milk*

Steps to Cook

1. Preheat the air fryer to 355 Fahrenheit. Add the flour, butter, salt, and milk to the bowl and knead the dough until smooth and refrigerate for 15-minutes.

2. Abode a frying pan over medium heat and add the oil to it. When the oil is heated, add the onions into the pan and sauté them. Improve spinach to pan and cook until it wilts. Drain excess moisture from spinach. Whisk the eggs together and add cheese to the bowl and mix.

3. Proceeds the dough out of the fridge and divides it into 8 equal parts. Roll the dough into a round that will fit into the bottom of the quiche mound. Place the rolled

dough into molds. Place the spinach filling over the dough. Place molds into air fryer basket and place basket inside of air fryer and cook for 15-minutes.

4. Remove quiche from molds and serve warm or cold

Avocado Toast with Tomato and Cottage Cheese

TIME TO PREPARE
5 minutes

COOK TIME
0 minutes

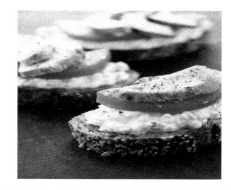

SERVING
2 People

Ingredients

- *½ cup cottage cheese*
- *½ avocado, mashed*
- *1 teaspoon Dijon mustard*
- *Dash hot sauce (optional)*
- *2 slices whole-grain bread, toasted*
- *2 slices tomato*

Steps to Cook

1. Mix together the cottage cheese, avocado, mustard, and hot sauce, if using, until well mixed in a small bowl.
2. Spread the mixture on the toast.
3. Top each piece of toast with a tomato slice.

Texas Toast Casserole

TIME TO PREPARE
5 minutes

COOK TIME
50 minutes

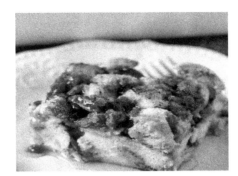

SERVING
4 People

Ingredients

- 1/2 cup butter, melted
- 1 cup brown Swerve
- 1 lb. Texas Toast bread, sliced
- 4 large eggs
- 1 1/2 cup milk
- 1 tablespoon vanilla extract
- 2 tablespoons Swerve
- 2 teaspoons cinnamon
- Maple syrup for serving

Steps to Cook

1. Layer a 9x13 inches baking pan with cooking spray. Spread the bread slices at the bottom of the prepared pan. Whisk the eggs with the remaining ingredients in a mixer. Pour this mixture over the bread slices evenly.

2. Bake the bread for 30 minutes at 350 degrees F in a preheated oven. Serve.

Banana Barley Porridge

TIME TO PREPARE
15 minutes

COOK TIME
5 minutes

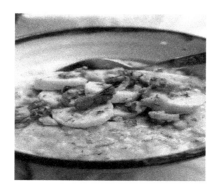

SERVING
2 People

Ingredients

- *1 cup divided unsweetened coconut milk*
- *1 small peeled and sliced banana*
- *1/2 cup barley*
- *3 drops liquid Stevia*
- *1/4 cup chopped coconuts*

Steps to Cook

1. In a bowl, properly mix barley with half the coconut milk and Stevia.
2. Cover the blending bowl, then refrigerate for about 6 hours.
3. In a saucepan, mix the barley mixture with coconut milk.
4. Cook for about 5 minutes on moderate heat.
5. Then top it with the chopped coconuts and, therefore, the banana slices.
6. Serve.

Cheese Omelette

TIME TO PREPARE
10 minutes

COOK TIME
15 minutes

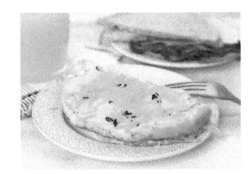

SERVING
2 People

Ingredients

- *3 eggs*
- *1 large yellow onion, diced*
- *2 tablespoons cheddar cheese, shredded*
- *½ teaspoon soy sauce*
- *Salt and pepper to taste*
- *Olive oil cooking spray*

Steps to Cook

1. In a container whisk together eggs, soy sauce, pepper, and salt. Spray with olive oil cooking spray a small pan that will fit inside of your air fryer. Swell onions to the pan and spread them around. Air fry onions for 7-minutes. Pour the beaten egg mixture over the cooked onions and sprinkle the top with shredded cheese. Abode back into the air fryer and cook for 6-minutes more.

2. Remove from the air fryer and serve Omelette with toasted multi-grain bread.

Wild Rice

TIME TO PREPARE
5 minutes

COOK TIME
2-3 hours

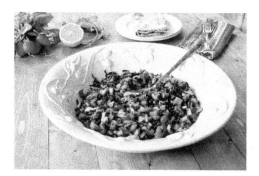

SERVING
2 People

Ingredients

- ¼ cup onions, diced
- ½ cup wild rice, or wild rice mixture, uncooked
- ¾ cups chicken broth, low sodium
- ¼ cup diced green or red peppers
- ⅛ teaspoon pepper
- ½ tablespoon oil
- ⅛ teaspoon salt
  - ¼ cup mushrooms, sliced

Steps to Cook

1. In a slow cooker, layer the rice and the vegetables and then pour oil, pepper, and salt over the vegetables. Stir well.
2. Heat the chicken broth in a pot, and then pour over the ingredients in the slow cooker.
3. Close the lid and cook for 2 ½-3 hours on high, until the rice has softened and the liquid is absorbed.
4. Serve and enjoy!

Zucchini Bread

TIME TO PREPARE
5 minutes

COOK TIME
40 minutes

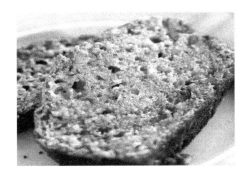

SERVING
4 People

Ingredients

- 3 eggs
- 1 1/2 cups Swerve
- 1 cup apple sauce
- 2 cups zucchini, shredded
- 1 teaspoon vanilla
- 2 cups flour
- 1/4 teaspoon baking powder
- 1 teaspoon baking soda
- 1 teaspoon cinnamon
- 1/2 teaspoon ginger
- 1 cup unsalted nuts, chopped

Steps to Cook

1. Thoroughly whisk the eggs with the zucchini, apple sauce, and the rest of the ingredients in a bowl.
2. Once mixed evenly, spread the mixture in a loaf pan. Bake it for 1 hour at 375 degrees F in a preheated oven. Slice and serve.

Bacon and Brussels Sprout Breakfast

TIME TO PREPARE
10 minutes

COOK TIME
15 minutes

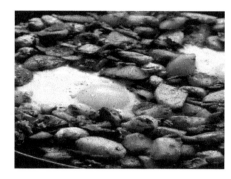

SERVING
3 People

Ingredients

- 1½ tablespoons Apple cider vinegar
- Salt
- 2 Minced shallots
- 2 Minced garlic cloves
- 3 medium eggs
- 12 oz. Black pepper Sliced Brussels sprouts
- 2 oz. Chopped bacon
- 1 tablespoon melted butter

Steps to Cook

1. Over medium heat, quickly fry the bacon until crispy, then reserve on a plate.
2. Set the pan ablaze again to fry garlic and shallots for 30 seconds.
3. Stir in apple vinegar, Brussels sprouts, and seasoning to cook for five minutes.
4. Add the bacon to cook for five minutes, then stir in the butter and set a hole in the middle.
5. Crash the eggs to the pan and let cook fully.
6. Enjoy.

Bagels

TIME TO PREPARE
50 minutes

COOK TIME
15 minutes

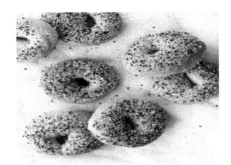

SERVING
12 People

Ingredients

- ½ lb. flour
- 1 tsp. Active dry yeast
- 1 tsp. Brown sugar
- ½ cup lukewarm water
- 2 tbsp. butter softened
- 1 tsp. salt
- 1 large egg

Steps to Cook

1. Liquefy the yeast and sugar in the warm water. Let rest for 5 minutes.
2. Add the remaining ingredients and mix until sticky dough forms. Cover, then let rest for 40 minutes.
3. Massage the dough on a lightly floured surface and divide into 5 large balls. Let rest for 4 minutes.
4. Preheat air fryer to 360 degrees F.
5. Flatted the dough balls and make a hole in the center of each. Arrange the bagels on a baking sheet lined with parchment paper—Bake for 20 minutes.
6. Enjoy!

TIME TO PREPARE
5 minutes

COOK TIME
15 minutes

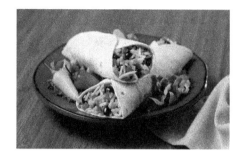

SERVING
2 People

Ingredients

- *1 Tablespoon Olive oil*
- *2 Corn tortillas*
- *¼ cup Red onion, chopped*
- *¼ cup Red bell peppers, chopped*
- *½, Red chili, deseeded and chopped*
- *2 Eggs*
- *Juice of 1 lime*
- *1Tablespoon Cilantro, chopped*

Steps to Cook

1. Turn the broiler to medium heat and place the tortillas underneath for 1 to 2 minutes on each side or until lightly toasted.

2. Remove and keep the broiler on.

3. Sauté onion, chili, and bell peppers for 5 to 6 minutes or until soft.

4. Place the eggs on top of the onions and peppers and place the skillet under the broiler for 5-6 minutes or until the eggs are cooked.

5. Serve half the eggs and vegetables on top of each tortilla and sprinkle with cilantro and lime juice to serve.

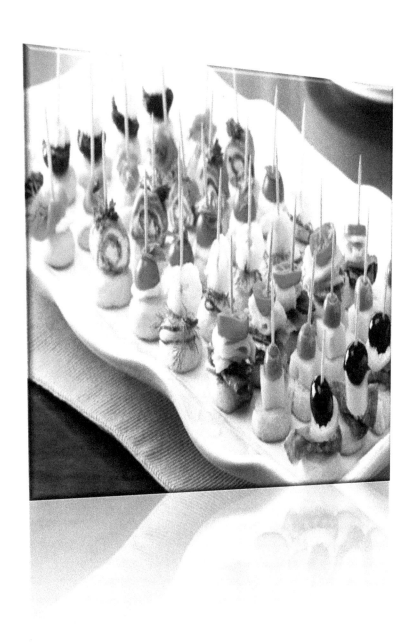

Appetizers & Snacks Recipes

Mortadella & Bacon Balls

TIME TO PREPARE
10 minutes

COOK TIME
30 minutes

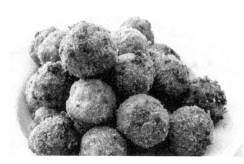

SERVING
2 People

Ingredients

- *4 ounces Mortadella sausage*
- *4 bacon slices, cooked and crumbled*
- *2 tbsp almonds, chopped*
- *½ tsp Dijon mustard*
- *3 ounces cream cheese*

Steps to Cook

1. Combine the mortadella and almonds in the bowl of your food processor. Pulse until smooth. Whisk the cream cheese and mustard in another bowl. Make balls out of the mortadella mixture.
2. Make a thin cream cheese layer over. Coat with bacon, arrange on a plate, and chill before serving.

Sheet Pan Chicken Fajita Lettuce Wraps

TIME TO PREPARE
15 minutes

COOK TIME
30 minutes

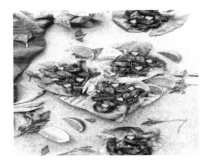

SERVING
2 People

Ingredients

- *1 lb. chicken breast, thinly sliced into strips*
- *2 teaspoons of olive oil*
- *2 bell peppers, thinly sliced into strips*
- *2 teaspoon of fajita seasoning*
- *6 leaves from a romaine heart*
- *Juice of half a lime*
- *¼ cup plain of non-fat Greek yogurt*

Steps to Cook

1. Preheat your oven to about 4000F.
2. Combine all of the ingredients apart from lettuce in a large bag, which will be resealed. Mix alright to coat vegetables and chicken with oil and seasoning evenly.
3. Spread the contents of the bag evenly on a foil-lined baking sheet. Bake it for about25-30 minutes, until the chicken is thoroughly cooked.
4. Serve on lettuce leaves and topped with Greek yogurt if you wish.

Onion Rings

TIME TO PREPARE
7 minutes

COOK TIME
10 minutes

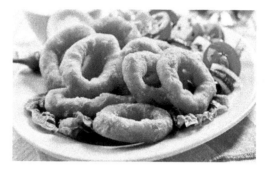

SERVING
3 People

Ingredients

- *1 onion, cut into slices then separate into rings*
- *1 ½ cups almond flour*
- *¾ cup pork rinds*
- *1 cup milk*
- *1 egg*
- *1 tablespoon baking powder*
- *½ teaspoon salt*

Steps to Cook

1. Preheat your air fryer for 10-minutes. Cut onion into slices, then separate into rings. In a container, supplement the flour, baking powder, and salt. Whisk the eggs, and the milk then combines with flour. Gently dip the floured onion rings into the batter to coat them.

2. Spread the pork rings on a plate and dredge the rings in the crumbs. Abode the onion rings in your air fryer and cook for 10-minutes at 360 Fahrenheit.

Crab & Spinach Dip

TIME TO PREPARE
10 minutes

COOK TIME
2 hours

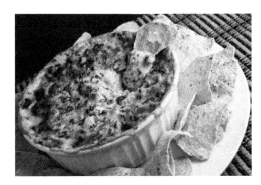

SERVING
10 People

Ingredients

- *1 pkg. frozen chopped spinach, thawed and squeezed nearly dry*
- *8 oz. reduced-fat cream cheese*
- *6 ½ oz. can crab meat, drained and shredded*
- *6 oz.jar marinated artichoke hearts, drained and diced fine*
- *¼ tsp hot pepper sauce*
- *Melba toast or whole-grain crackers (optional)*

Steps to Cook

1. Remove any shells or cartilage from the crab.
2. Place all ingredients in a small crockpot. Cover and cook on high 1 ½ - 2 hours, or until heated through and cream cheese is melted. Stir after 1 hour.
3. Serve with Melba toast or whole-grain crackers. The serving size is ¼ cup.

Seasoned Pita Chips

TIME TO PREPARE
5 minutes

COOK TIME
10 minutes

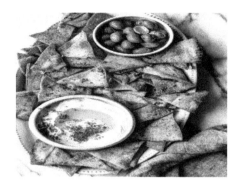

SERVING
2 People

Ingredients

- 3 whole-grain pitas with pitas
- 3 tablespoons of seasoning from Italy
- 1 chili powder teaspoon
- 1 teaspoon of powdered garlic
- 1 salt teaspoon

Steps to Cook

1. Preheat the oven to 425 degrees. Coat the cooking spray with a baking sheet.
2. Halve the pitas, stack all 6 halves, and split the pitas into 6 wedges. Spread the wedges over the baking sheet on the soft side. Sprinkle with a skinny coat of cooking spray and spices.
3. Place in the oven and cook until browned and crisp, for 5-10 minutes.

Caprese Skewers

TIME TO PREPARE
5 minutes

COOK TIME
0 minutes

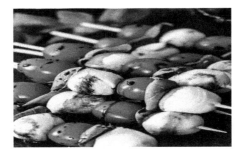

SERVING
2 People

Ingredients

- *12 cherry tomatoes*
- *12 basil leaves*
- *8 (1-inch) pieces mozzarella cheese*
- *¼ cup Italian Vinaigrette (optional, for serving)*

Steps to Cook

1. On each of 4 wooden skewers, thread the following: 1 tomato, 1 basil leaf, 1 piece of cheese, 1 tomato, 1 basil leaf, 1 piece of cheese, 1 basil leaf, 1 tomato.
2. Serve with the vinaigrette, if desired, for dipping.

Charred Bell Peppers

TIME TO PREPARE
7 minutes

COOK TIME
4 minutes

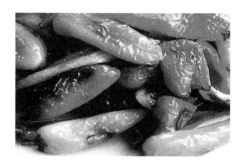

SERVING
3 People

Ingredients

- *20 bell peppers, sliced and seeded*
- *1 teaspoon olive oil*
- *1 pinch of sea salt*
- *1 lemon*

Steps to Cook

1. Preheat your air fryer to 390 Fahrenheit. Sprinkle the peppers with oil and salt. Cook the peppers in the air fryer for 4-minutes. Place peppers in a large bowl, and squeeze lemon juice over the top. Season with salt and pepper.

Cinnamon Apple Chips

TIME TO PREPARE
5 minutes

COOK TIME
10 minutes

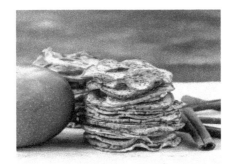

SERVING
2 People

Ingredients

- 1 medium apple, sliced thin
- ¼ tsp cinnamon
- ¼ tsp nutmeg
- Nonstick cooking spray

Steps to Cook

1. Heat oven to 375. Spray a baking sheet with cooking spray. Place apples in a mixing bowl and add spices. Toss to coat.
2. Arrange apples, in a single layer, on the prepared pan. Bake 4 minutes, turn apples over, and bake 4 minutes more.
3. Serve immediately.

Maple Pumpkin Nutrition Bars

TIME TO PREPARE
10 minutes

COOK TIME
18 minutes

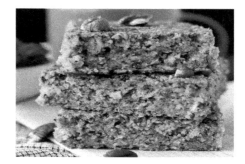

SERVING
4 People

Ingredients

- 1 (15 ounces) can drained and rinsed, Great Northern beans
- 1/2 cup of purée with pumpkin
- 4 teaspoons of sugar with maple
- 1 pumpkin pie spice teaspoon
- 1/4 of a teaspoon of salt
- 1 cup of cereal with raisin bran
- Vanilla whey protein powder for 6 scoops
- Old-fashioned oats with 1 1/2 cups
- 1 spelled flour cup

Steps to Cook

1. Preheat the oven to 350 degrees.
2. Place all the ingredients except the oats and flour in a food processor or blender. Blend until the ingredients are smooth, then pour dry and pulse until just mixed.
3. In vegetable oil, gently coat a 9×13-inch baking dish and spread the mixture out evenly.
4. Place in the oven and bake until set, or for 15-18 minutes. Remove and slice through 10 bars.

Garlic Kale Chips

TIME TO PREPARE
5 minutes

COOK TIME
15 minutes

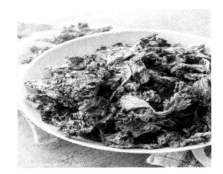

SERVING
2 People

Ingredients

- 1 (16 oz.) bunch kale, trimmed and cut into 2-inch pieces
- 2 tablespoons extra-virgin olive oil
- 1 teaspoon sea salt
- ½ teaspoon garlic powder
- Pinch cayenne (optional, to taste)

Steps to Cook

1. Preheat the oven to 350°F, then line two baking sheets with parchment paper.
2. Wash the kale and pat it completely dry.
3. In a large bowl, toss the kale with olive oil, sea salt, garlic powder, and cayenne, if using.
4. Spread the kale in a single layer on the prepared baking sheets.
5. Bake until crisp, 12 to 15 minutes, rotating the sheets once.

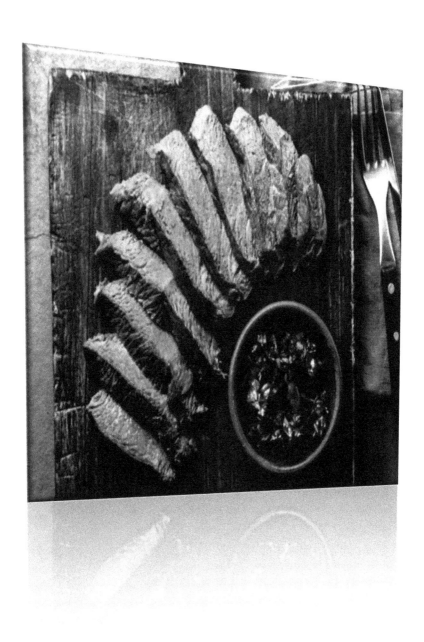

Meat Recipes

Lemon and Honey Pork Tenderloin

TIME TO PREPARE
5 minutes

COOK TIME
10 minutes

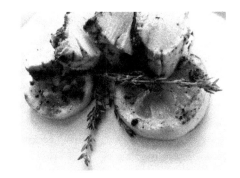

SERVING
4 People

Ingredients

- *1 (1-pound / 454-g) pork tenderloin, cut into ½-inch slices*
- *1 tablespoon olive oil*
- *1 tablespoon freshly squeezed lemon juice*
- *1 tablespoon honey*
- *½ teaspoon grated lemon zest*
- *½ teaspoon dried marjoram*
- *Pinch salt*
- *Freshly ground black pepper, to taste*

Steps to Cook

1. Put the pork tenderloin in a medium bowl.
2. In a minor bowl, combine the olive oil, lemon juice, honey, lemon zest, marjoram, salt, and pepper. Mix.
3. Pour this marinade over the tenderloin slices and massage gently with your hand to work it into the pork.
4. Place the pork in the air fryer basket and roast at 400ºF (204ºC) for 10 minutes or until the pork registers at least 145ºF (63ºC) using a meat thermometer.

Asparagus Beef Sauté

TIME TO PREPARE
10 minutes

COOK TIME
30 minutes

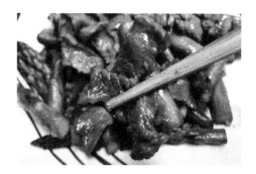

SERVING
4 People

Ingredients

- *1 lb. beef tenderloin or sirloin, trimmed and sliced*
- *12 oz. asparagus*
- *1 carrot, peeled and shredded*
- *1 teaspoon crushed herbes de Provence*
- *¼ teaspoon lemon peel, grated*
- *½ cup marsala wine*
- *2 teaspoons olive oil*
- *Cooked rice*
- *Salt and pepper to taste*

Steps to Cook

1. Cut into 2-inch pieces. Heat oil over medium temperature in your skillet.
2. Now cook the carrot, beef, pepper, and salt for 3 minutes. Keep stirring. Add the herbes de Provence and asparagus. Cook for 2 more minutes.
3. Add the lemon peel and marsala. Bring down the heat. Cook for 5 minutes uncovered.
4. Serve with cooked rice.

Black-Eyed Peas with Greens & Pork

TIME TO PREPARE
10 minutes

COOK TIME
30 minutes

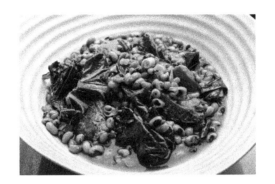

SERVING
2 People

Ingredients

- *1 pound of boneless, trimmed pork chops, cut into 1/2- inch sections*
- *1/2 teaspoon salt, break*
- *1/4 of a freshly ground teaspoon of pepper*
- *1 tablespoon of oil with canola*
- *1 onion medium, chopped*
- *2 tablespoons of paste for tomatoes*
- *Instant brown rice for 1 cup*
- *8 cups of finely chopped kale leaves, tough stems separated*

Steps to Cook

1. Toss pork with 1/4 teaspoon salt and pepper, then heat oil over medium heat in a large nonstick skillet. Add the pork and cook for 4 to six minutes, stirring, until cooked thoroughly, and move with a slotted spoon to a bowl.

2. Add onion, ingredient, and rice to the pan and cook for about 4 minutes before the onion softens.

3. Add kale and garlic and cook for 1 to 2 minutes before the kale begins to wilt.

4. Stir in water, vinegar, paprika, and therefore the remaining 1/4 teaspoon salt. Bring back a boil.

5. Cover, reduce heat, and simmer for 15 to twenty minutes until the rice is completed. Put in the reserved pork

(about 1 small bunch)
- *Garlic 4 cloves, minced*
- *1 (14.1 ounces) sodium chicken broth will decrease*
- *2 teaspoons of vinegar for cider, or sherry vinegar smoke paprika with 1/2 teaspoon, preferably hot*
- *1 (15 ounces) can be rinsed with black-eyed peas*

and black-eyed peas and warmth for 1 minute.

Pork Chop Diane

TIME TO PREPARE
10 minutes

COOK TIME
20 minutes

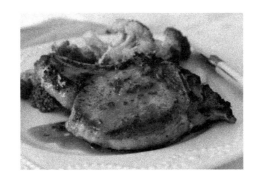

SERVING
2 People

Ingredients

- *8 cup low-sodium chicken broth*
- *½ tablespoon freshly squeezed lemon juice*
- *1 teaspoon Worcestershire sauce*
- *1 teaspoon Dijon mustard*
- *2 (5 oz.) boneless pork top loin chops*
- *½ teaspoon extra-virgin olive oil*
- *½ teaspoon lemon zest*
- *½ teaspoon butter*
- *1 teaspoon chopped fresh chives*

Steps to Cook

1. Blend together the chicken broth, lemon juice, Worcestershire sauce, and Dijon mustard and set it aside.
2. Season the pork chops lightly.
3. Situate a large skillet over medium-high heat and add the olive oil.
4. Cook the pork chops, turning once, until they are no longer pink, about 8 minutes per side.
5. Put aside the chops.
6. Pour the broth mixture into the skillet and cook until warmed through and thickened, about 2 minutes.
7. Blend lemon zest, butter, and chives.
8. Garnish with a generous spoonful of sauce.

Beef Korma Curry

TIME TO PREPARE
10 minutes

COOK TIME
17-20 minutes

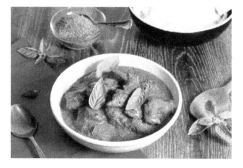

SERVING
4 People

Ingredients

- *1 pound (454 g) sirloin steak, sliced*
- *½ cup yogurt*
- *1 tablespoon curry powder*
- *1 tablespoon olive oil*
- *1 onion, chopped*
- *2 cloves garlic, minced*
- *1 tomato, diced*
- *½ cup frozen baby peas, thawed*

Steps to Cook

1. In a medium bowl, combine the steak, yogurt, and curry powder. Stir and set aside.
2. In a metal bowl, combine the olive oil, onion, and garlic. Bake at 350ºF (177ºC) for 3 to 4 minutes or until crisp and tender.
3. Add the steak along with the yogurt and the diced tomato. Bake for 12 to 13 minutes or until the steak is almost tender.
4. Stir in the peas and bake for 2 to 3 minutes or until hot.

Beef Bourguignon Stew

TIME TO PREPARE
10 minutes

COOK TIME
30 minutes

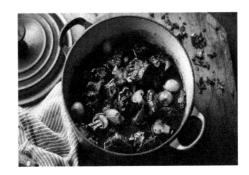

SERVING
6 People

Ingredients

- 1 tbsp. butter or olive oil 1½ lbs. diced stewing meat
- 4 slices bacon, sliced
- 1 small white onion, diced
- 1 clove garlic, crushed
- 2 stalks celery, sliced
- 8 oz. mushrooms, sliced
- 1 cup low-sodium beef stock
- 1 cup good-quality dry red wine
- 2 tbsp. tomato paste
- 1 bay leaf
- ½ tsp. dried thyme

Steps to Cook

1. Select the "Sauté" function on your Instant Pot and sauté the bacon until crispy.

2. Once done, set aside and reserve the bacon grease in the pot.

3. Sear the beef in the Instant Pot, working in batches to avoid overcrowding the pot and stewing the beef.

4. Discard all but a tablespoon of the drippings from the pot, and add a tablespoon of butter or preferred cooking oil.

5. Sauté the onions and celery to the pot, until soft, and then add the mushrooms. Stir in the garlic, then cook for one minute.

6. Remove all the vegetables and set them aside on a side plate.

- *½ tsp. xanthan gum*
- *½ tsp. sea salt, or to taste)*
- *¼ tsp. freshly ground black pepper*
- *1 tbsp. fresh parsley chopped*

7. Add xanthan gum to the Instant Pot, followed by the wine; deglaze the pot thoroughly.

8. Simmer until the wine begins to thicken, and then add the beef broth.

9. Stir in the tomato paste, bay leaf, and thyme, and simmer until the sauce is sufficiently reduced.

10. Return the sautéed vegetables, beef, and bacon to the pot, then stir in the salt and black pepper.

11. Cover and seal the Instant Pot, making sure the steam release handle is pointed to "Sealing."

12. Select the "Meat/Stew" function and adjust it to cooking for 30 minutes. Once done, do a quick pressure release and uncover the stew.

13. Taste and adjust for seasoning, remove and discard the bay leaf and garnish with parsley prior to serving.

Creamy Paprika Pork

TIME TO PREPARE
10 minutes

COOK TIME
25 minutes

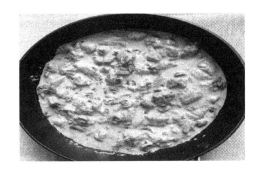

SERVING
2 People

Ingredients

- *18 ounces of boneless skinless pork loin or breast of chicken*
- *Strong quality ground paprika with 4 teaspoons*
- *1 Tablespoon (or salt, pepper, garlic, and onion) Stacey Hawkins Splash of Desperation Seasoning*
- *1/2-1 Tablespoon of Roasted Garlic Oil Stacey Hawkins*
- *Greek Yogurt, 12 ounces, simple, unflavored*
- *1/2-1 Tablespoon Stacey Hawkins*

Steps to Cook

1. Cut the meat into 1-inch pieces and put them in a big tub.
2. Sprinkle seasonings with paprika and Dash of Desperation with beef. Toss to cover completely.
3. In a large skillet, add the roasted garlic oil and cook over medium-high heat.
4. Add the meat to the pan and cook, until browned, for 5-7 minutes. Stir occasionally.
5. Garlic and onion, and yogurt are added to the pan. Reduce heat to medium and bring to a simmer.
6. Simmer the meat for 3-5 minutes before the liquid decreases slightly to make a thicker sauce and thoroughly cook the chicken. Stir occasionally.

Garlic and Spring Onion

- *4 Cups of plain cauliflower rice, steamed (optional)*

7. Divide the cauliflower rice into four equal servings and portion over 1 C.

Lamb Shoulder

TIME TO PREPARE
10 minutes

COOK TIME
30 minutes

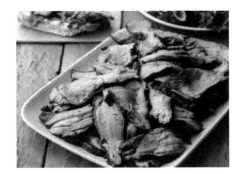

SERVING
62 People

Ingredients

- 2 tsp. good olive oil
- 4 lbs. bone-in lamb shoulder
- 2 cups low-sodium beef or chicken stock
- 1 sprig of fresh rosemary
- 6 chopped anchovies
- 1 tsp. garlic purée
- 1 tsp. dried oregano
- 1 1/2 tsp. Kosher salt

Steps to Cook

1. Select the "Sauté" function on your Instant Pot and add oil.
2. Once hot, add the lamb shoulder and sear until nicely browned. Set aside for now.
3. Add the chicken stock to deglaze the bottom of the pan and then stir in the anchovies and garlic.
4. Return the lamb to the Instant Pot insert, sprinkle with salt and oregano, and then add the rosemary sprig.
5. Cover and seal the Instant Pot, turning the pressure valve to "Sealing." Cook on the "Manual, High Pressure" setting for 1½ hours.
6. Once done, allow for a 15-minute natural pressure release and then

do a quick pressure release to release any remaining steam.

7. Slice and serve with your favorite side.

Lemon Greek Beef and Vegetables

TIME TO PREPARE
10 minutes

COOK TIME
20 minutes

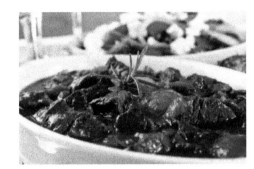

SERVING
4 People

Ingredients

- *½ pound (227 g) 96% lean ground beef*
- *2 medium tomatoes, chopped*
- *1 onion, chopped*
- *2 garlic cloves, minced*
- *2 cups fresh baby spinach*
- *2 tablespoons freshly squeezed lemon juice*
- *1/3 cup low-sodium beef broth*
- *2 tablespoons crumbled low-sodium feta cheese*

Steps to Cook

1. In a baking pan, crumble the beef. Place in the air fryer basket. Air fry at 370ºF (188ºC) for 3 to 7 minutes, stirring once during cooking until browned. Drain off any fat or liquid.
2. Swell the tomatoes, onion, and garlic into the pan. Air fry for 4 to 8 minutes more, or until the onion is tender.
3. Add the spinach, lemon juice, and beef broth.
4. Air fry for 2 to 4 minutes more, or until the spinach is wilted. Sprinkle with the feta cheese and serve immediately.

Buffalo Chicken Tenders

TIME TO PREPARE
15 minutes

COOK TIME
6 minutes

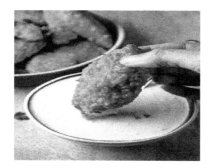

SERVING
4 People

Ingredients

- 1 pound chicken fillet
- ½ cup pork rinds
- 4 oz Parmesan, grated
- ½ tsp ground black pepper
- 1 tbsp olive oil
- 2 eggs, whisked
- ½ teaspoon salt
- 1/3 cup Buffalo sauce

Steps to Cook

1. In the mixing bowl, mix up together pork rinds with grated cheese.
2. Cut the chicken fillet into medium size tenders.
3. Sprinkle the poultry with ground black pepper and salt.
4. Dip every chicken tender in the whisked eggs and coat in the pork rind mixture.
5. Pour olive oil into the pan and preheat it.
6. Add the chicken tenders and cook them for 2-3 minutes from each side or until the chicken tenders are light brown.
7. Dry the chicken tenders with the help of the paper towel if needed and transfer them to the serving plate.

Provencal Ribs

TIME TO PREPARE
10 minutes

COOK TIME
30 minutes

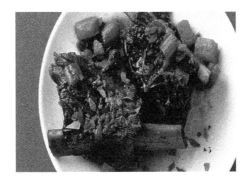

SERVING
4 People

Ingredients

- *500g of pork ribs*
- *Provencal herbs*
- *Salt*
- *Ground pepper*
- *Oil*

Steps to Cook

1. Put the ribs in a bowl and add some oil, Provencal herbs, salt, and ground pepper.
2. Stir well and leave in the fridge for at least 1 hour.
3. Put the ribs in the basket of the air fryer and select 2000C for 20 minutes. From time to time, shake the basket and remove the ribs.

Orange Chicken

TIME TO PREPARE
5 minutes

COOK TIME
30 minutes

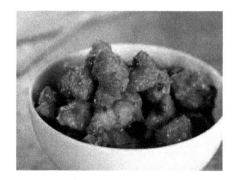

SERVING
4 People

Ingredients

- *1 lb. of skinless, boneless chicken, cut into bites*
- *1/2 tsp Crystal Light drink in orange*
- *1 tsp of powdered garlic*
- *Dried ground ginger with 1/2 tsp*
- *1/4 TL red flakes of pepper*
- *1/8 teaspoon pepper*
- *2 Teaspoons of olive oil*
- *2 Tbsp of vinegar for rice*
- *Water 2 tbsp*
- *1/2 teaspoon of sesame oil*

Steps to Cook

1. Preheat the 350-degree oven to
2. In a 13"x9 "baking dish, put the chicken.
3. In a small cup, the remaining ingredients are missing. Pour chicken over it. Bake until done, for 25-30 minutes.

- *1 teaspoon of medium soy sauce*
- *1/2 Tbsp of minced dried onion*
- *1/4-1/2 tsp of orange peel dried*

Doner Kebabs

TIME TO PREPARE
10 minutes

COOK TIME
35 minutes

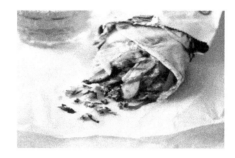

SERVING
2 People

Ingredients

- *1 egg, lightly beaten*
- *250g 10% fat minced lamb*
- *1 teaspoon ground cinnamon*
- *half teaspoon ground cumin*
- *1 heaped tsp oregano*
- *half teaspoon chili flakes*
- *grated zest and juice half lemon*
- *half slice wholemeal bread, crumbled*
- *good pinch of white pepper*
- *Juice half lemon, to serve*
- *2 cloves garlic, crushed*

Steps to Cook

1. In a mixing bowl, combine the oregano, cinnamon, cumin, chili, pepper, garlic, lemon zest, and juice, as well as the egg and crumbled bread.
2. With a fork, thoroughly combine the ingredients, breaking up the bread even further.
3. In a separate bowl, combine the lamb and set aside for 10 minutes. Mix again, then form into a loaf with a diameter of 6cm and a length of 13.5cm. Cook Allow to cool for 5 minutes before slicing thinly and stuffing into pita bread with salad.
4. Serve with a squeeze of lemon juice.

- *4 wholemeal pitta bread (70grams each)*
- *4 large servings salad (cucumber, 100g iceberg lettuce, 300grams tomatoes, and 150grams red onion)*

Pork Burgers with Red Cabbage Slaw

TIME TO PREPARE
20 minutes

COOK TIME
9 minutes

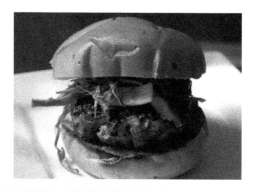

SERVING
4 People

Ingredients

- ½ cup Greek yogurt
- 2 tablespoons low-sodium mustard, divided
- 1 tablespoon freshly squeezed lemon juice
- ¼ cup sliced red cabbage
- ¼ cup grated carrots
- 1 pound (454 g) lean ground pork
- ½ teaspoon paprika
- 1 cup mixed baby lettuce greens
- 2 small tomatoes, sliced
- 8 small low-sodium whole-

Steps to Cook

1. In a lesser bowl, syndicate the yogurt, 1 tablespoon mustard, lemon juice, cabbage, and carrots; mix and refrigerate.

2. In a medium bowl, combine the pork, the remaining 1 tablespoon mustard, and paprika. Form into 8 small patties.

3. Lay the patties into the air fryer basket. Air fry at 400ºF (204ºC) for 7 to 9 minutes, or until the patties register 165ºF (74ºC) as tested with a meat thermometer.

4. Assemble the burgers by placing some of the lettuce greens on a bun bottom. Top with a tomato slice, the patties, and the cabbage mixture.

wheat sandwich buns, cut in half

5. Add the bun top and serve immediately.

Kielbasa (Polish Sausage) With Cabbage and Potatoes

TIME TO PREPARE
30 minutes

COOK TIME
8 hours

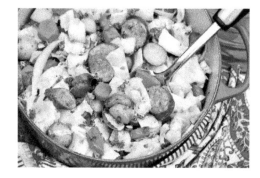

SERVING
2 People

Ingredients

- ½ lb Kielbasa, sliced into rings
- 2 cups Green Cabbage, sliced into thin strips
- 1 small, diced Potato
- 1 small finely diced Onion
- ¼ of a tsp. Caraway Seeds
- ¼ of a tsp. Sea Salt
- 6oz Chicken Stock r

Steps to Cook

1. Place everything in your crockpot and stir to mix.
2. Cook, covered, on low for 10 hours, then serve.

Root Beer Pork

**TIME TO
PREPARE**
10 minutes

COOK TIME
30 minutes

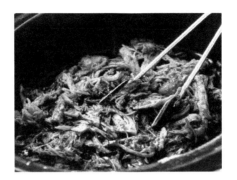

SERVING
2 People

Ingredients

- *1 lb. Pork roast*
- *Black pepper*
- *6 c sliced Onion*
- *3 c Root beet*
- *2 T Ketchup*
- *1.5 tsp Almond flour*
- *25 tsp Lemon juice*
- *1.5 tsp Worcestershire sauce*
- *1 T Tomato paste*
- *1.5 tsp Honey*

Steps to Cook

1. Season roast with pepper and garlic salt, and put in the pot. Mix the rest of the ingredients together, then pour on the roast. Lock and seal the lid.
2. Set to meat/stew for 35 minutes. Carefully release pressure Take out onions and roast.
3. Discard the onions and shred the pork and stir the pork back into the pot.

Salsa Lime Chicken

TIME TO PREPARE
10 minutes

COOK TIME
45 minutes

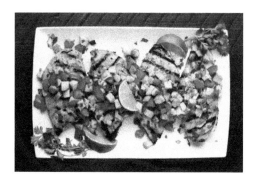

SERVING
4 People

Ingredients

- *5 boneless, skinless breasts of chicken*
- *4 tablespoons of lime juice,*
- *1 1/4 tablespoons of chili powder*
- *1 1/4 of a cup of salsa fresh*

Steps to Cook

1. Preheat the oven to 350 ° C.
2. Line the foil with a 13X9 baking dish. Spray with non-stick cooking spray.
3. Put the chicken in your baking dish. Sprinkle the powder with chili. Add juice from lime. Great with salsa.
4. Bake until done, for 40-45 minutes.

Chicken Squash and Coriander Pilaf

TIME TO PREPARE
10 minutes

COOK TIME
30 minutes

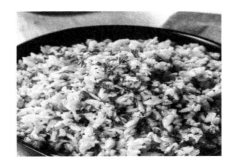

SERVING
4 People

Ingredients

- *2 teaspoon sunflower oil*
- *250 g/9 oz wholegrain rice, rinsed in several changes of water, then drained*
- *2 teaspoon mild curry powder*
- *1 teaspoon ground cumin*
- *1 teaspoon ground coriander*
- *1/2 teaspoon ground turmeric*
- *2 tablespoon flaked almonds*
- *750 ml/26 fl oz water*
- *1 yellow or green courgette, thinly sliced*

Steps to Cook

1. Preheat the oven to 180°C (160° fan)/350°F/gas mark 4 and heat the sunflower oil until hot in an ovenproof casserole or baking dish placed over medium heat.
2. Stir in the rice and cook for 2 minutes in the oil, stirring frequently. Cook for an additional 2-3 minutes, or until the spices are fragrant.
3. Cover with water and stir thoroughly. Before placing the squash and chicken on top of the rice, bring to a boil.
4. Cover the dish loosely with aluminum foil and bake for about 28 minutes, or until the rice has absorbed the liquid and the chicken is cooked through.

- *Freshly ground black pepper*
- *2 large skinless chicken breasts (400g), trimmed of excess fat*
- *1/2 lemon, juiced*
- *1 handful coriander leaves*

5. Remove the foil from the oven and set it aside.

6. Return the dish to the oven for an additional 8-10 minutes, or until the almonds are golden brown.

7. Remove the baking sheet from the oven. Place the chicken on a plate and set aside for 5 minutes to cool before shredding with two forks.

8. To separate the grains, add some lemon juice to the pilaf and fluff the rice with a fork.

9. Until serving, top with the shredded chicken and some coriander leaves.

Greek Lamb Pita Pockets

TIME TO PREPARE
15 minutes

COOK TIME
5-7 minutes

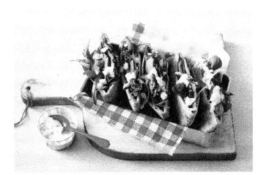

SERVING
4 People

Ingredients

- *Dressing:*
- *1 cup plain Greek yogurt*
- *1 tablespoon lemon juice*
- *1 teaspoon dried dill weed, crushed*
- *1 teaspoon ground oregano*
- *½ teaspoon salt*
- *Meatballs:*
- *½ pound (227 g) ground lamb*
- *1 tablespoon diced onion*
- *1 teaspoon dried parsley*
- *1 teaspoon dried dill weed, crushed*
- *¼ teaspoon oregano*

Steps to Cook

1. Stir dressing ingredients together and refrigerate while preparing lamb.

2. Combine all meatball ingredients in a large bowl and stir to distribute seasonings.

3. Shape meat mixture into 12 small meatballs, rounded or slightly flattened if you prefer.

4. Air fry at 390ºF (199ºC) for 5 to 7 minutes, until well done. Remove and drain on paper towels.

5. To serve, pile meatballs and your choice of toppings in pita pockets and drizzle with dressing.

- ¼ teaspoon coriander
- ¼ teaspoon ground cumin
- ¼ teaspoon salt
- 4 pita halves
- Suggested Toppings:
- Red onion, slivered
- Seedless cucumber, thinly sliced
- Crumbled feta cheese
- Sliced black olives
- Chopped fresh peppers

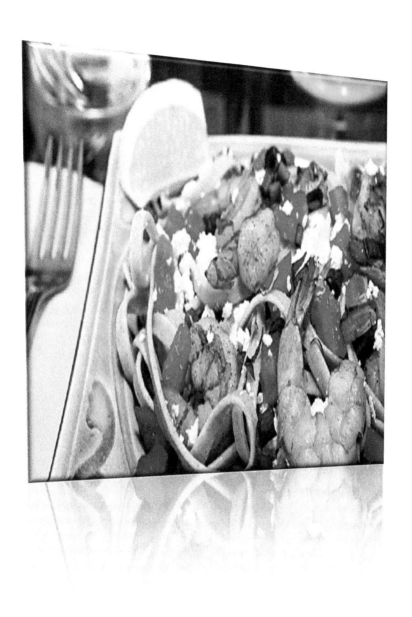

Fish & Seafood Recipes

Avocado Orange Salmon

TIME TO PREPARE
10 minutes

COOK TIME
15 minutes

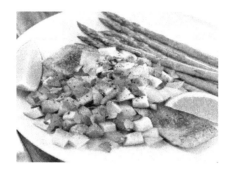

SERVING
8 People

Ingredients

- About 3 cups watercress, roughly chopped
- 3 tbsp cucumbers, finely chopped
- 4 (4–6 ounces each) Alaska salmon fillets, rinsed and dried
- ¼ cup avocado oil (divided)
- 2 oranges, peeled and segmented, discard membranes
- 1 tsp white wine vinegar
- Salt and pepper to taste

Steps to Cook

1. Heat 3 tablespoons of avocado oil over medium heat in a medium saucepan or skillet.
2. Add the salmon and brown evenly for 3–4 minutes.
3. Flip the salmon and season with salt and pepper; cook for 3–4 more minutes until opaque.
4. Divide onto serving plates.
5. Add the watercress, cucumber, and orange segments to a mixing bowl; mix well.
6. Add the remaining oil, white wine vinegar, salt, and pepper.
7. Add the mixture to the serving plates beside the salmon, top with apple cider vinegar, avocado, and walnuts.

- *½ avocado, pitted, peeled, and sliced*
- *2 cups mixed greens*
- *¼ cup walnuts*
- *2 tbsp apple cider vinegar*
- *1 pinch smoked paprika*

Mussels in Tomato Sauce

TIME TO PREPARE
10 minutes

COOK TIME
30 minutes

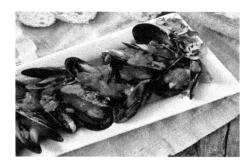

SERVING
4 People

Ingredients

- 2 tomatoes, seeded and chopped finely
- 2 pounds mussels, scrubbed and de-bearded
- 1 cup low-sodium chicken broth
- 1 tablespoon fresh lemon juice
- 2 garlic cloves, minced r

Steps to Cook

1. In the pot of Instant Pot, place tomatoes, garlic, wine, and bay leaf and stir to combine.
2. Arrange the mussels on top.
3. Close the lid and place the pressure valve in the "Seal" position.
4. Press "Manual" and cook under "High Pressure" for 3 minutes. Press "Cancel" and carefully allow a "Quick" release.
5. Open the lid and serve hot.

Garlic Shrimp Zucchini Noodles

**TIME TO
PREPARE**
12 minutes

COOK TIME
4 minutes

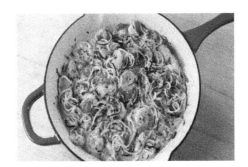

SERVING
5 People

Ingredients

- *16 ounces uncooked shrimps, shelled and deveined*
- *1 tablespoon olive oil*
- *1 cup cherry tomatoes, cut in half*
- *8 cups zucchini strips*
- *2 tablespoons minced garlic*
- *1 teaspoon dried oregano*
- *½ teaspoon chili powder*
- *½ teaspoon salt*

Steps to Cook

1. Brush the shrimps with vegetable oil. Place on a skillet and cook for two minutes on all sides or until pink. Set aside.

2. Place the remainder of the ingredients in a bowl and add the shrimps.

3. Season with salt, then toss to coat the ingredients.

Quick Shrimp Scampi

TIME TO PREPARE
10 minutes

COOK TIME
8 minutes

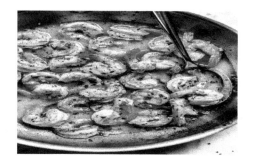

SERVING
2 People

Ingredients

- 30 (1 pound / 454 g) uncooked large shrimp, peeled, deveined, and tails
- removed
- 2 teaspoons olive oil
- 1 garlic clove, thinly sliced Juice, and zest of ½ lemon
- 1/8 teaspoon kosher salt
- Pinch of red pepper flakes (optional)
- 1 tablespoon chopped fresh parsley

Steps to Cook

1. Sprig a baking pan with nonstick cooking spray, then combine the shrimp, olive oil, sliced garlic, lemon juice and zest, kosher salt, and red pepper flakes (if using) in the pan, tossing to coat. Place in the air fryer basket.

2. Roast at 360ºF (182ºC) for 7 to 8 minutes or until firm and bright pink.

3. Remove the fryer's shrimp, place on a serving plate, and sprinkle the parsley on top. Serve warm.

Crunchy Crusted Salmon

TIME TO PREPARE
10 minutes

COOK TIME
15 minutes

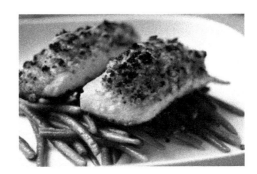

SERVING
4 People

Ingredients

- 2 slices whole-wheat bread, torn into pieces
- 4 teaspoons honey
- 2 teaspoons canola oil
- 3 tablespoons finely chopped walnuts 4 (4-ounce) salmon fillets
- 4 teaspoons Dijon mustard
- ½ teaspoon dried thyme

Steps to Cook

1. Preheat the oven to 400°F (200°C). Grease a baking sheet with some cooking spray.
2. Place the salmon over the baking sheet.
3. Combine the mustard and honey in a bowl, brush the salmon with the honey mixture.
4. Add the bread pieces to a blender or food processor and blend them to make fine crumbs.
5. Add the crumbs and walnuts to a mixing bowl. Mix well.
6. Add the thyme and canola oil; combine again.
7. Press the mixture over the salmon and bake for 12–15 minutes until the topping is evenly brown and the salmon is easy to flake. Serve warm.

Parmesan Herb Fish

TIME TO PREPARE
10 minutes

COOK TIME
30 minutes

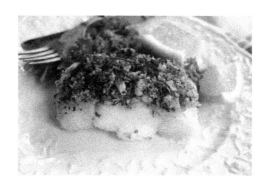

SERVING
4 People

Ingredients

- 16 oz. tilapia fillets
- 1/3 cup almonds, sliced and chopped
- ½ teaspoon parsley, chopped
- ¼ cup dry bread crumbs
- ½ teaspoon garlic powder
- ¼ teaspoon black pepper, ground
- ½ teaspoon paprika
- 3 tablespoons Parmesan cheese, grated
- Olive oil

Steps to Cook

1. Preheat your oven to 350 ºF.
2. Mix the bread crumbs, almonds, seasonings, and Parmesan cheese in a dish. Brush oil lightly on the fish.
3. Coat the almond mix evenly.
4. Now keep the fish on a greased foil-lined baking pan.
5. Bake for 10-12 minutes. The fish should flake easily with your fork.

Salmon Stew

TIME TO PREPARE
8 minutes

COOK TIME
12 minutes

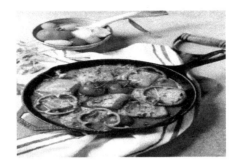

SERVING
2 People

Ingredients

- 1 pound salmon fillet, sliced
- 1 onion, chopped
- Salt, to taste
- 1 tablespoon butter, melted
- 1 cup fish broth
- ½ teaspoon red chili powder

Steps to Cook

1. Season the salmon fillets with salt and red flavoring.
2. Put butter and onions in a skillet and sauté for about 3 minutes.
3. Add seasoned salmon and cook for about 2 minutes on all sides.
4. Add fish broth and secure the lid.
5. Cook for about 7 minutes on medium heat and open the lid.
6. Dish out and serve immediately.
7. Transfer the stew to a bowl and put it aside to cool for meal prepping. Divide the mixture into 2 containers. Cover the containers and refrigerate for about 2 days. Reheat in the microwave before serving.

Fish Tacos

TIME TO PREPARE
15 minutes

COOK TIME
12 minutes

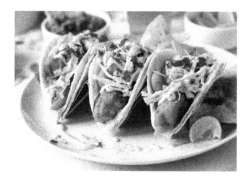

SERVING
4 People

Ingredients

- 1 pound (454 g) white fish fillets, such as snapper
- 1 tablespoon olive oil
- 3 tablespoons freshly squeezed lemon juice, divided
- 1½ cups chopped red cabbage
- ½ cup of salsa
- 1/3 cup sour cream
- 6 whole-wheat tortillas
- 2 avocados, peeled and chopped

Steps to Cook

1. Skirmish the fish with olive oil and sprinkle with 1 tablespoon of lemon
2. juice. Place in the air fryer basket and air fry at 400ºF (204ºC) meant for 9 to 12 minutes or until the fish just flakes when tested with a fork.
3. Meanwhile, combine the remaining 2 tablespoons of lemon juice, cabbage, salsa, and sour cream in a medium bowl.
4. As momentarily as the fish is cooked, remove it from the air fryer basket and break it into large pieces.
5. Let everyone assemble their taco combining the fish, tortillas, cabbage mixture, and avocados.

Cajun Shrimp & Roasted Vegetables

TIME TO PREPARE
10 minutes

COOK TIME
30 minutes

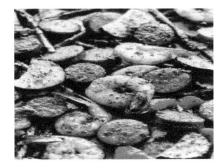

SERVING
4 People

Ingredients

- *1 lb. large shrimp, peeled and deveined*
- *2 zucchinis, sliced*
- *2 yellow squash, sliced*
- *½ bunch asparagus, cut into thirds*
- *2 red bell pepper, cut into chunks*
- *2 tbsp. olive oil*
- *2 tbsp. Cajun Seasoning*
- *Salt & pepper, to taste*

Steps to Cook

1. Heat oven to 400 degrees.
2. Combine shrimp and vegetables in a large bowl. Add oil and seasoning and toss to coat.
3. Spread evenly in a large baking sheet and bake 15-20 minutes, or until vegetables are tender. Serve.

Asian-Inspired Swordfish Steaks

TIME TO PREPARE
10 minutes

COOK TIME
10 minutes

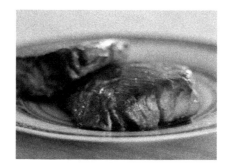

SERVING
4 People

Ingredients

- 4 (4-ounce / 113-g) swordfish steaks
- ½ teaspoon toasted sesame oil
- 1 jalapeño pepper, finely minced
- 2 garlic cloves, grated
- 1 tablespoon grated fresh ginger
- ½ teaspoon Chinese five-spice powder
- 1/8 teaspoon freshly ground black pepper
- 2 tablespoons freshly squeezed lemon juice

Steps to Cook

1. Place the swordfish steaks on a work surface and drizzle with the sesame oil.

2. In a small bowl, mix the jalapeño, garlic, ginger, five-spice powder, pepper, and lemon juice. Rub this mixture into the fish and let it stand for 10 minutes. Put in the air fryer basket.

3. Roast at 380ºF (193ºC) for 6 to 11 minutes, or until the swordfish reaches an inner temperature of at least 140ºF (60ºC) on a meat thermometer. Serve immediately.

Sesame-Crusted Tuna with Green Beans

TIME TO PREPARE
15 minutes

COOK TIME
5 minutes

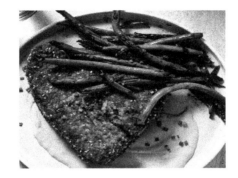

SERVING
4 People

Ingredients

- 1/4 cup white sesame seeds
- 1/4 cup black sesame seeds
- 4 (6-ounce) ahi tuna steaks
- Salt and pepper
- 1 tablespoon olive oil
- 1 tablespoon coconut oil
- 2 cups green beans

Steps to Cook

1. In a shallow dish, mix the two kinds of sesame seeds.
2. Season the tuna with pepper and salt.
3. Dredge the tuna in a mixture of sesame seeds.
4. Heat up to high heat the olive oil in a skillet, then add the tuna.
5. Cook for 1 to 2 minutes until it turns seared, then sear on the other side.
6. Remove the tuna from the skillet and let the tuna rest while using the coconut oil to heat the skillet.
7. Fry the green beans in the oil for 5 minutes then use sliced tuna to eat.

Paprika Butter Shrimp

TIME TO PREPARE
15 minutes

COOK TIME
15 minutes

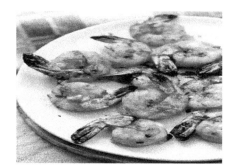

SERVING
2 People

Ingredients

- ¼ tablespoon smoked paprika
- 1/8 cup sour cream
- ½ pound shrimp
- 1/8 cup butter
- Salt and black pepper, to taste

Steps to Cook

1. Preheat the oven to 390 degrees and grease a baking dish.
2. Place in the oven and bake for about a quarter-hour.
3. Place paprika shrimp in a dish and put aside to chill for meal prepping.
4. Divide it into 2 containers and cover the lid. Refrigerate for 1-2 days, then reheat in microwave before serving.

Ranch Tilapia fillets

TIME TO PREPARE
7 minutes

COOK TIME
17 minutes

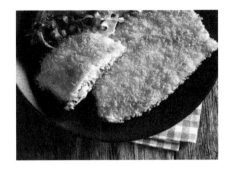

SERVING
2 People

Ingredients

- *2 tablespoons flour*
- *1 egg, lightly beaten*
- *1 cup crushed cornflakes*
- *2 tablespoons ranch seasoning*
- *2 tilapia fillets*
- *Olive oil spray*

Steps to Cook

1. Place a parchment liner in the air fryer basket, then scoop the flour out onto a plate; set it aside.
2. Put the beaten egg in a medium shallow bowl.
3. Abode the cornflakes in a zip-top bag and crush with a rolling pin or another small, blunt object.
4. On another plate, mix to combine the crushed cereal and ranch seasoning.
5. Dredge the tilapia fillets in the flour, then dip in the egg, and then press into the cornflake mixture.
6. Place the prepared fillets on the liner in the air fryer in a single layer.
7. Spray lightly with olive oil, and air fry at 400ºF (204ºC) for 8 minutes. Carefully flip the fillets and spray

with more oil. Air fry for an additional 9 minutes, until golden and crispy, and serve.

Crab Curry

TIME TO PREPARE
10 minutes

COOK TIME
30 minutes

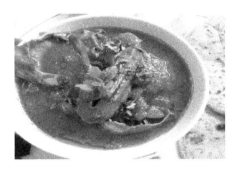

SERVING
2 People

Ingredients

- *0.5lb chopped crab*
- *1 thinly sliced red onion*
- *0.5 cup chopped tomato*
- *3tbsp curry paste*
- *1tbsp oil or ghee*

Steps to Cook

1. Set the Instant Pot to saute and add the onion, oil, and curry paste. When the onion is soft, add the remaining ingredients and seal.
2. Cook on Stew for 20 minutes. Release the pressure naturally.

Chilean Sea Bass with Green Olive Relish

TIME TO PREPARE
10 minutes

COOK TIME
20 minutes

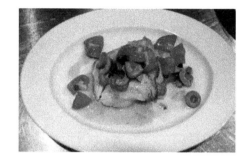

SERVING
4 People

Ingredients

- Olive oil spray
- 2 (6-ounce / 170-g) Chilean sea bass fillets or other firm-fleshed white fish
- 3 tablespoons extra-virgin olive oil
- ½ teaspoon ground cumin
- ½ teaspoon kosher salt
- ½ teaspoon black pepper
- 1/3 cup pitted green olives, diced
- ¼ cup finely diced onion
- 1 teaspoon chopped capers

Steps to Cook

1. Spray the air fryer basket with olive oil spray. Drizzle the fillets with olive oil, then sprinkle with the cumin, salt, and pepper. Abode the fish in the air fryer basket. Bake at 325ºF (163ºC) for 10 minutes, or until the fish flakes easily with a fork.

2. In the meantime, in a lesser bowl, stir together the olives, onion, and capers and serve the fish topped with the relish.

Seafood Salad with Avocado

TIME TO PREPARE
10 minutes

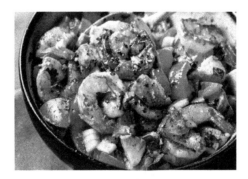

SERVING
4 People

COOK TIME
5 minutes

Ingredients

- 6 oz shrimps, peeled
- 5 oz smoked salmon, roughly chopped
- 1 avocado, chopped
- 1 tbsp avocado oil
- 1 tsp pumpkin seeds
- ½ tsp cayenne pepper
- ½ cup lettuce
- 1 tsp lemon juice
- ½ tsp turmeric

Steps to Cook

1. Preheat oven to 420°F/215°C. Blend the first five ingredients. Sprinkle potato with 2 tbsps. of this mixture. Bake for 20 minutes.
2. Sprinkle fillets with the remaining mixture and add to the potatoes. Cook for about 15 minutes and serve.

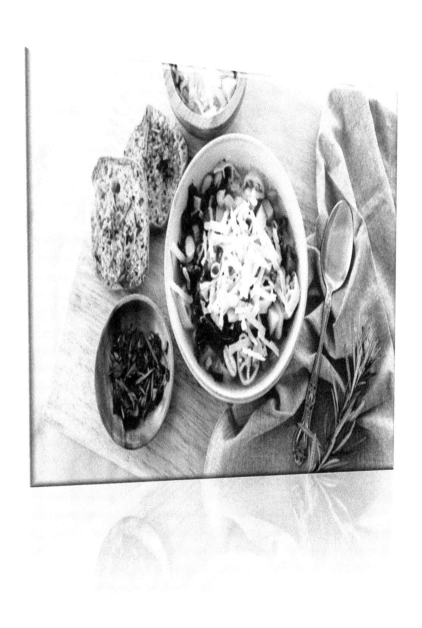

Soup & Salad Recipes

Crockpot Veggies Soup

TIME TO PREPARE
5 minutes

COOK TIME
4-6 hours

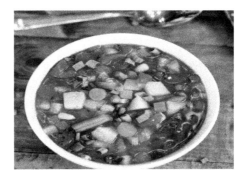

SERVING
2 People

Ingredients

- 1 garlic clove, minced
- 4 ⅔ oz. tomatoes, diced, with juice
- 1 celery stalks, diced
- 2 cups vegetable broth, low-sodium
- ⅓ large onion, diced
- 1 cup cabbage, chopped
- 1 large carrot, diced
- ⅓ teaspoon Spike seasoning, salt-free
- ⅓ large sweet potato, peeled & diced
- Salt, optional

Steps to Cook

1. In a crockpot, stir all the ingredients together, and then set the pot on high.
2. Allow cooking for about 4-6 hours.
3. When through, stir gently and then mash parsnips and sweet potatoes lightly in order to slightly thicken the soup.
4. Serve and enjoy!

- *⅓ medium parsnip, diced*
- *Black pepper*
- *⅓ red bell pepper, seeded & diced*

Avocado and Caprese Salad

TIME TO PREPARE
15 minutes

COOK TIME
19 minutes

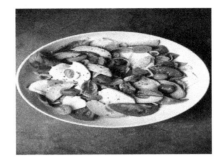

SERVING
6 People

Ingredients

- *2 avocados, cubed*
- *1 cup cherry tomatoes, halved*
- *8 ounces cashew cheese*
- *2 tablespoons finely chopped fresh basil*
- *2 tablespoons olive oil*
- *2 tablespoons balsamic vinegar*
- *1 tablespoon salt*
- *Fresh ground black pepper*

Steps to Cook

1. Take a bowl and add the listed Ingredients: toss them well until thoroughly mixed
2. Season with pepper consistent with your taste
3. Serve and enjoy!

French Onion Soup

TIME TO PREPARE
10 minutes

COOK TIME
1 hours 15 minutes

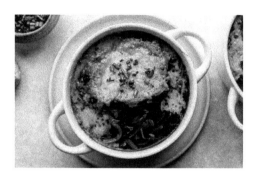

SERVING
4 People

Ingredients

- 1 teaspoon low-salt soy sauce
- 3 teaspoons sunflower oil
- 400grams sweet potatoes (cut into 12 wedges)
- 1 low-salt vegetable stock cube, dissolved in 800ml boiled water
- 20grams reduced-fat mature Cheddar cheese
- 20grams mozzarella
- 1 tablespoon fresh parsley, finely chopped, plus extra to serve

Steps to Cook

1. Preheat the oven to 190 degrees Celsius/gas 5.
2. In a saucepan, heat 2 teaspoons of the oil, then add the onions and cook, stirring constantly, for 30–40 minutes, until the onions caramelize.
3. Place the remaining oil on a baking sheet while the onions are caramelizing. Muddle the potatoes in the mixture until they are
4. evenly coated, then bake for 30–35 minutes.
5. Add the stock to the onions, bring to a boil, and then reduce to low heat for 5 minutes.
6. Meanwhile, to make the cheesy croutons: Grill each half-slice of bread, then turn over and top with

- *1kilogram onions, finely chopped*
- *4 slices wholemeal bread (30grams per slice)*
- *Good pinch of pepper*

the Cheddar cheese and mozzarella, then grill until the cheese melts and browns.

7. Alternatively, place the cheese-topped bread on a baking sheet and bake for 5-10 minutes.

8. Pour the soup into four bowls and stir in the parsley, pepper, and soy sauce.

9. Serve with sweet potato wedges on the side, as well as cheesy croutons and a sprinkling of fresh parsley on top.

Broccoli and Mushroom Salad

TIME TO PREPARE
10 minutes

COOK TIME
40 minutes

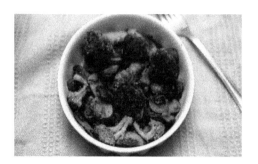

SERVING
4 People

Ingredients

- 4 sun-dried tomatoes, cut in half
- 3 cup torn leaf lettuce
- 1 ½ cup broccoli florets
- 1 cup mushrooms, sliced 1/3 cup radishes, sliced
- What you'll need from the store cupboard: 2 tbsp. water
- 1 tbsp. balsamic vinegar 1 tsp vegetable oil
- ¼ tsp chicken bouillon granules
- ¼ tsp parsley
- ¼ tsp dry mustard

Steps to Cook

1. Place tomatoes in a small bowl and pour boiling water over, just enough to cover. Let stand 5 minutes, drain.
2. Chop tomatoes and place in a large bowl. Add lettuce, broccoli, mushrooms, and radishes.
3. In a jar with a tight-fitting lid, add the remaining ingredients and shake well.
4. Pour over salad and toss to coat.
5. Serve.

- *1/8 tsp cayenne pepper*

Classic Split Pea Soup

TIME TO PREPARE
5 minutes

COOK TIME
6-8 hours

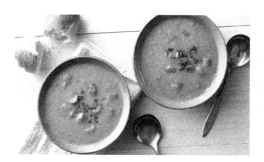

SERVING
2 People

Ingredients

- ½ cup celery, chopped
- 8 oz. split peas, dried
- 1 ½ cups water
- 1 carrot, chopped
- ¼ teaspoon salt
- ½ cup onion, chopped
- ¼ teaspoon pepper
- ½ cup ham, low-sodium, diced, cooked
- 2 cups chicken broth, low sodium

Steps to Cook

1. To a slow cooker, add peas along with the remaining ingredients.
2. Close the lid and allow to cook for 8 hours on low until the peas have become tender and the soup has thickened.
3. When through, remove the bay leaf and discard it.
4. Ladle the pea soup to the bowls and then serve immediately. Enjoy!

Ginger Soup

TIME TO PREPARE
10 minutes

COOK TIME
10 minutes

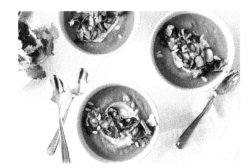

SERVING
4 People

Ingredients

- *1 Can Diced Tomatoes*
- *1 Can Peppers*
- *6 cups Vegetable Broth*
- *3 Cups Green Onions, Diced*
- *2 Cups Mushrooms, Sliced*
- *3 Teaspoons Garlic, minced*
- *3 Teaspoons Ginger, Fresh & Grated*
- *4 Tablespoons Tamari*
- *2 Cups Bok Choy, Chopped*
- *1 Tablespoon Cilantro, Chopped*

Steps to Cook

1. Add all ingredients apart from your carrot and scallion into a saucepan, then bring it to a boil using medium-high heat.
2. Lower to medium-low, cooking for 6 minutes.
3. Stir in your carrots and green onions, cooking for an additional two minutes.
4. Serve with cilantro.

- *3 Tablespoons Carrot Grated*

Roasted Chicory and Orange Salad

TIME TO PREPARE
10 minutes

COOK TIME
30 minutes

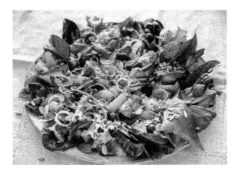

SERVING
2 People

Ingredients

- *1 teaspoon fresh thyme or pinch dried*
- *Freshly ground black pepper*
- *4 heads chicory, halved lengthways*
- *Grated rind and juice 1 orange*
- *1 teaspoon olive oil*
- *2 oranges, segmented*
- *2 teaspoons orange zest, to garnish*

Steps to Cook

1. Preheat the oven to 200 degrees Celsius/gas 6.
2. In an ovenproof bowl, position the chicory. Combine the orange rind and juice, oil, and thyme in a mixing bowl. Season with plenty of black pepper and sprinkle over the chicory.
3. Cook for 28-30 minutes, or until they are tender and starting to char.
4. Toss with the orange segments and serve with some cooking liquid and orange zest drizzled on top. Allow to cool slightly or chill before serving.

Ham Hock Soup

TIME TO PREPARE
10 minutes

COOK TIME
30 minutes

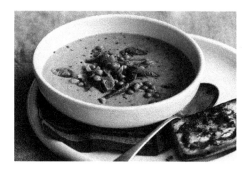

SERVING
2 People

Ingredients

- *1 lb. ham hock on the bone*
- *1 lb. green peas*
- *1 cup vegetable broth*
- *1 cup shredded cabbage and onion*
- *1 tbsp. mixed herbs*

Steps to Cook

1. Mix all the ingredients in your Instant Pot, cook on Stew for 10 minutes. Release the pressure naturally and serve.

Mushroom Stew

TIME TO PREPARE
7 minutes

COOK TIME
1 hour 22 minutes

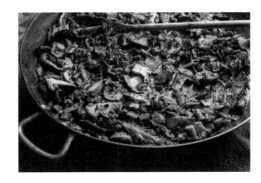

SERVING
6 People

Ingredients

- *1 lb. Of chicken, cubed, boneless, skinless*
- *2 tablespoons of canola oil*
- *1 lb. Fresh mushrooms, sliced*
- *1 tablespoon thyme, dried*
- *¾ cup of water*
- *2 tablespoons tomato paste*
- *3 large tomatoes, chopped*
- *4 cloves garlic, minced*
- *1 cup green peppers, sliced*
- *3 cups of zucchini, diced*

Steps to Cook

1. Cut the chicken into cubes.
2. Position them in the air fryer basket and pour olive oil over them.
3. Add mushrooms, zucchini, onion, and green pepper.
4. Mix and add in garlic, cook for 2-minutes, then add in tomato paste, water, and seasonings.
5. Lock the air fryer and cook the stew for 50-minutes.
6. Set the heat to 340 Fahrenheit and cook for an additional 20-minutes.
7. Remove from air fryer and transfer into a large pan.
8. Empty in a bit of water and simmer for 10-minutes.

- *1 large onion, diced*
- *1 tablespoon basil*
- *1 tablespoon marjoram*
- *1 tablespoon oregano*

Bean Salad with Balsamic Vinaigrette

TIME TO PREPARE
5 minutes

COOK TIME
0 minutes

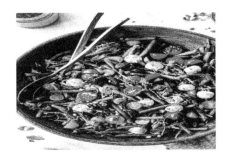

SERVING
2 People

Ingredients

- *For the Vinaigrette:*
- *2 tablespoons balsamic vinegar*
- *⅓ cup fresh parsley, chopped*
- *4 garlic cloves, finely chopped*
- *Ground black pepper, to taste*
- *¼ cup Extra-virgin olive oil*
- *For the Salad:*
- *⅓ can (15 oz.) low-sodium garbanzo beans, rinsed and drained*
- *⅓ can (15 oz.) low-sodium black beans, rinsed and drained*

Steps to Cook

1. In a small pan, mix the balsamic vinegar, parsley, garlic, and pepper to prepare the vinaigrette. Slowly add the olive oil when whisking.

2. In a large pan, combine the beans and the onion.

3. Pour the vinaigrette over the mixture and stir softly, blend thoroughly and coat equally. Cover and refrigerate.

4. Put one lettuce leaf on each plate to serve. Divide the salad between the individual plates and garnish with the minced celery. Serve straight away.

- *1 small red onion, diced*
- *2 lettuce leaves*
- *Celery, finely chopped*

Chickpea and Tuna Salad

TIME TO PREPARE
10 minutes

COOK TIME
0 minutes

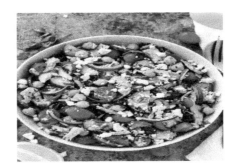

SERVING
2 People

Ingredients

- 20ml extra-virgin olive oil
- 2 lemon wedges
- grated zest half a lemon
- 150grams salad leaves/lettuce pinch black pepper
- 1 small red onion, finely chopped
- 1 x 400grams tin chickpeas in water, drained (drained weight 240grams)
- 180grams ripe cherry tomatoes, cut into quarters
- 8cm cucumber, chopped

Steps to Cook

1. In a large mixing bowl, combine the lemon zest, pepper, and olive oil; add the red onion, tomatoes, and cucumber; mix well, and set aside for a few minutes to infuse.

2. Fold in the chickpeas and tuna gently so that it is evenly covered in the dressing.

3. Finally, add the salad leaves and split between two lunch boxes, along with a lemon wedge to squeeze over the top before eating.

- *1 x 200grams tin tuna in water, drained (drained weight 150grams)*

Zucchini "Pasta" Salad

TIME TO PREPARE
10 minutes

COOK TIME
40 minutes

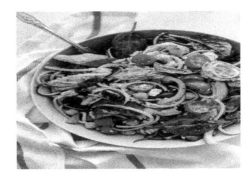

SERVING
5 People

Ingredients

- 5 oz. zucchini, spiralized
- 1 avocado, peeled and sliced
- 1/3 cup feta cheese, crumbled
- ¼ cup tomatoes, diced
- ¼ cup black olives, diced
- 1/3 cup Green Goddess Salad Dressing
- 1 tsp olive oil
- 1 tsp basil
- Salt and pepper to taste

Steps to Cook

1. Place zucchini on a paper towel-lined cutting board. Sprinkle with a little bit of salt and let sit for 30 minutes to remove excess water. Squeeze gently.

2. Add oil to medium skillet, then heat over med-high heat. Add zucchini and cook, stirring frequently, until soft, about 3 – 4 minutes.

3. Transfer zucchini to a large bowl, then add remaining ingredients, except for the avocado. Cover and chill for 1 hour.

4. Serve topped with avocado.

Prosciutto Spinach Salad

TIME TO PREPARE
5 minutes

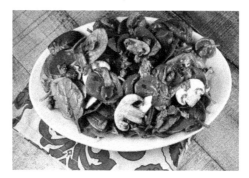

SERVING
2 People

COOK TIME
5 minutes

Ingredients

- *2 cups baby spinach*
- *1/3 lb. prosciutto*
- *1 cantaloupe*
- *1 avocado*
- *¼ cup diced red onion handful of raw, unsalted walnuts*

Steps to Cook

1. Put a cup of spinach on each plate.
2. Top with the diced prosciutto, cubes of melon balls, slices of avocado, a couple of purple onions, and a couple of walnuts.
3. Add some freshly ground pepper if you wish.
4. Serve!

Squash Soup

TIME TO PREPARE
5 minutes

COOK TIME
4 hours 10 minutes

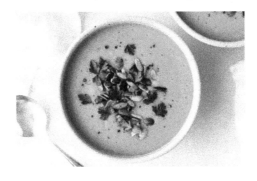

SERVING
2 People

Ingredients

- 1 garlic clove, minced
- 1 sprigs thyme
- 1 small onion, chopped
- 1 small butternut squash, peeled, cut into large cubes
- 1 small carrot, peeled, chopped
- ⅓ sprig sage
- Kosher salt & freshly ground pepper, to taste
- 1 cup chicken or vegetable broth, low sodium
- Cayenne, a pinch
- Freshly chopped parsley, to garnish

Steps to Cook

1. Combine the butternut squash together with carrot, garlic, onion, sage, and thyme in a slow cooker. Then pour in the broth along with salt, cayenne, and pepper to season.
2. Close the lid and cook for 8 hours on low or 4 hours on high, until the squash has become very tender.
3. When through, remove the herbs sprigs and transfer the soup into a blender. Blend the soup until smooth.
4. Stir in the heavy cream and then garnish with chopped parsley.
5. Serve and enjoy!

- *Heavy cream, to serve*

Watermelon and Arugula Salad

TIME TO PREPARE
10 minutes

COOK TIME
40 minutes

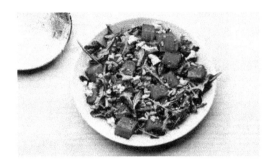

SERVING
6 People

Ingredients

- 4 cups watermelon, cut in 1-inch cubes
- 3 cup arugula
- 1 lemon, zested
- ½ cup feta cheese, crumbled
- ¼ cup fresh mint, chopped
- 1 tbsp. fresh lemon juice
- 3 tbsp. olive oil
- Fresh ground black pepper
- Salt to taste

Steps to Cook

1. Combine oil, zest, juice, and mint in a large bowl. Stir together.
2. Add watermelon and gently toss to coat. Add remaining ingredients and toss to combine. Taste and adjust seasoning as desired.
3. Cover and chill at least 1 hour before serving.

Salad of Eggless Eggs

TIME TO PREPARE
10 minutes

COOK TIME
0 minutes

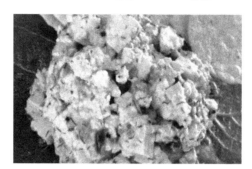

SERVING
2 People

Ingredients

- Vegenaise 2 Teaspoons
- The sweet relish of 1 tablespoon
- 1 teaspoon white vinegar distilled
- 1 teaspoon mustard
- 1/4 teaspoon Stevia or some other sweetener of natural origin
- 1/2 teaspoon turmeric from the field
- 1/4 dried dill teaspoon
- 1 tablespoon of parsley that's dried
- 1/8 teaspoon of salt

Steps to Cook

1. Combine the vegenaise, relish, vinegar, mustard, Stevia, turmeric, dill, parsley, salt, and pepper in a medium-sized bowl and blend well.

2. Add the tofu, onion, and celery to a separate bowl and toss to blend. In the vegenaise combination, pour the tofu mixture and blend until well mixed.

3. Until serving, refrigerate for at least 2 hours to let the flavors blend.

- *1/4 black pepper ground teaspoon*
- *1 pound of dried and crumbled extra-firm low-fat tofu*
- *1 spoon of chopped onion*
- *2 tablespoons celery chopped*

Chargrilled Vegetable Salad

TIME TO PREPARE
10 minutes

COOK TIME
10 minutes

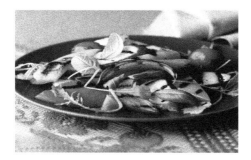

SERVING
2 People

Ingredients

- *3 tablespoon olive oil*
- *2 red pepper*
- *1 teaspoon of red wine vinegar*
- *1 aubergine*
- *2 red onion sliced*
- *1 red chili*
- *1 small garlic clove ground*
- *Plump sundried tomatoes in oil*
- *Handful black olive*
- *Large black basil, roughly torn*

Steps to Cook

1. Directly over the flame, blackened the pepper all over. Place them in a tub, cover with a plate, and set aside to cool fully.

2. In a big mixing bowl, combine the oil, vinegar, garlic, and chill.

3. Chargrill the onions, aubergine, and courgette in batches on a hot griddle pan until they have grill marks on both sides and are softening. The time limit is unquestionably determined by the temperature of your grill.

4. Put the vegetables in the dressing to marinate as soon as they're ready, breaking up the onions into rings.

5. Peel the peppers, cut the stalk, and scrape out the seeds when they are

cool enough to handle. Slice into strips and toss with the vegetables in the bowl's juice.

Pumpkin Spice Soup

TIME TO PREPARE
10 minutes

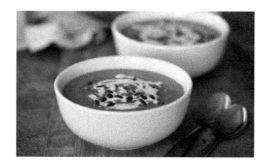

COOK TIME
30 minutes

SERVING
2 People

Ingredients

- *1lb cubed pumpkin*
- *1 cup low sodium vegetable broth*
- *2 tbsp mixed spice*

Steps to Cook

1. Mix all the ingredients in your Instant Pot. Cook on Stew for 35 minutes.
2. Release the pressure naturally. Blend the soup.

Broccoli Stilton Soup

TIME TO PREPARE
10 minutes

COOK TIME
35 minutes

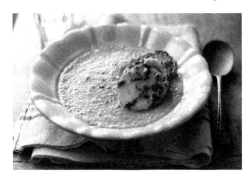

SERVING
2 People

Ingredients

- *1lb chopped broccoli*
- *0.5lb chopped vegetables*
- *1 cup low sodium vegetable broth*
- *1 cup Stilton*

Steps to Cook

1. Mix all the ingredients in your Instant Pot. Cook on Stew for 35 minutes.
2. Release the pressure naturally. Blend the soup.

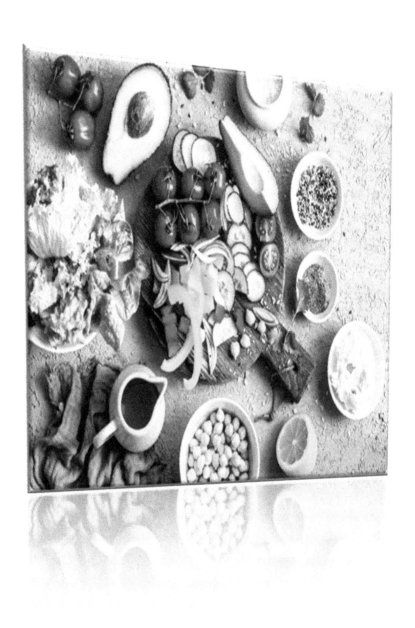

Vegetarian recipes

Three-Cheese Stuffed Mushrooms

TIME TO PREPARE
15 minutes

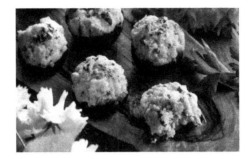

SERVING
3 People

COOK TIME
10 minutes

Ingredients

- *9 large button mushrooms, stems removed*
- *1 tablespoon olive oil*
- *Salt and ground black pepper, to taste*
- *1/2 teaspoon dried rosemary*
- *6 tablespoons Swiss cheese shredded*
- *6 tablespoons Romano cheese, shredded 6*
- *tablespoons cream cheese*
- *1 teaspoon soy sauce*
- *1 teaspoon garlic, minced*

Steps to Cook

1. Brush the mushroom caps with olive oil; sprinkle with salt, pepper, and rosemary.
2. In a mixing bowl, thoroughly combine the remaining ingredients, combine it well, and divide the filling mixture among the mushroom caps.
3. Cook in the preheated Air Fryer at 390 degrees F for 7 minutes. Let the mushrooms cool slightly before serving. Bon appétit!

- *3 tablespoons green onion, minced*

Onion and Zucchini Platter

TIME TO PREPARE
15 minutes

COOK TIME
45 minutes

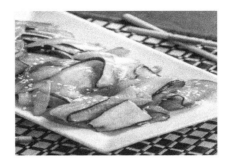

SERVING
4 People

Ingredients

- *3 large zucchinis, julienned*
- *1 cup cherry tomatoes, halved*
- *1/2 cup basil*
- *2 red onions, thinly sliced*
- *1/4 teaspoon salt*
- *1 teaspoon cayenne pepper*
- *2 tablespoons lemon juice*

Steps to Cook

1. Create zucchini noodles by employing a vegetable peeler and shaving the zucchini with a peeler lengthwise until you get to the core and seeds
2. Turn zucchini and repeat until you have long strips.
3. Discard seeds.
4. Lay strips on a chopping board and slice lengthwise to your required thickness.
5. Mix noodles in a bowl alongside onion, basil, tomatoes, and toss.
6. Sprinkle salt and cayenne pepper on top. Drizzle juice.
7. Serve and enjoy!

Potato and Lentil Curry

TIME TO PREPARE
10 minutes

COOK TIME
35 minutes

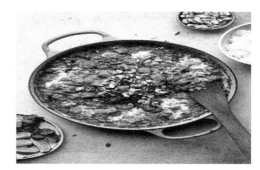

SERVING
2 People

Ingredients

- 1 teaspoon sunflower oil
- 1 onion, chopped
- 1 teaspoon mustard seeds
- 1 teaspoon chili powder
- 1 teaspoon ground coriander pinch turmeric
- 6 tablespoon fresh coriander, leaves, and finely chopped stalks
- 200g chopped tomatoes
- 2 tablespoon tomato purée
- 2cm fresh ginger, peeled and grated

Steps to Cook

1. In a medium saucepan, heat the sunflower oil.
2. Fry for 3 minutes after adding the onion.
3. Continue to fry for 1 minute after adding the mustard seeds, ginger, chili powder, coriander, turmeric, and fresh coriander.
4. Pour the stock over the tomatoes, tomato puree, and lentils in the pan.
5. Bring to a boil, then reduce heat to low, cover, and cook for 25-30 minutes, or until lentils are almost tender.
6. Stir in the potatoes and cook for another 10-15 minutes, or until they are tender.

- *125g yellow lentils, washed and drained*
- *600ml vegetable stock*
- *900g floury potatoes, peeled and cubed*
- *fresh coriander leaves, to serve*

7. Serve with raita made from yogurt and coriander leaves.

Eggplant Parmesan

TIME TO PREPARE
20 minutes

COOK TIME
15 minutes

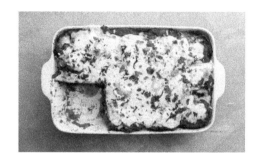

SERVING
4 People

Ingredients

- *1/2 cup and 3 tablespoons almond flour, divided*
- *1.25-pound eggplant, ½-inch sliced*
- *1 tablespoon chopped parsley*
- *1 teaspoon Italian seasoning*
- *2 teaspoons salt*
- *1 cup marinara sauce 1*
- *egg, pastured*
- *1 tablespoon water*
- *3 tablespoons grated parmesan cheese, reduced-fat*
- *1/4 cup grated mozzarella*

Steps to Cook

1. Slice the eggplant into ½-inch pieces, place them in a colander, sprinkle with 1 ½ teaspoon salt on both sides, and let it rest for 15 minutes.

2. Meanwhile, place ½ cup flour in a bowl, add egg and water and whisk until blended.

3. Place remaining flour in a shallow dish, add remaining salt, Italian seasoning, and parmesan cheese, and stir until mixed.

4. Switch on the air fryer, insert fryer basket, grease it with olive oil, then shut with its lid, set the fryer at 360 degrees F, and preheat for 5 minutes.

5. Meanwhile, drain the eggplant pieces, pat them dry, and then dip

cheese, reduced-fat

each slice into the egg mixture and coat with flour mixture.

6. Open the fryer, add coated eggplant slices in it in a single layer, close with its lid and cook for 8 minutes until nicely golden and cooked, flipping the eggplant slices halfway through the frying.

7. Then top each eggplant slice with a tablespoon of marinara sauce and some of the mozzarella cheese and continue air frying for 1 to 2 minutes or until cheese has melted.

8. When the air fryer beeps, open its lid, transfer eggplants onto a serving plate, and keep them warm.

9. Cook remaining eggplant slices in the same manner and serve.

Balsamic Root Vegetables

TIME TO PREPARE
25 minutes

COOK TIME
10 minutes

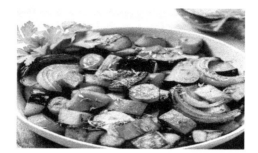

SERVING
3 People

Ingredients

- *2 potatoes, cut into 1 1/2-inch piece*
- *2 carrots, cut into 1 1/2-inch piece*
- *2 parsnips, cut into 1 1/2-inch piece*
- *1 onion, cut into 1 1/2-inch piece*
- *Pink Himalayan salt and ground black pepper, to taste*
- *1/4 teaspoon smoked paprika*
- *1 teaspoon garlic powder*
- *1/2 teaspoon dried thyme*
- *1/2 teaspoon dried marjoram*

Steps to Cook

1. Toss all ingredients in a large mixing dish.
2. Roast in the preheated Air Fryer at 400 degrees F for 10 minutes. Shake the basket and cook for 7 minutes more.
3. Serve with some extra fresh herbs if desired. Bon appétit!

- *2 tablespoons olive oil*
- *2 tablespoons balsamic vinegar*

Asparagus Frittata Recipe

TIME TO PREPARE
20 minutes

COOK TIME
20 minutes

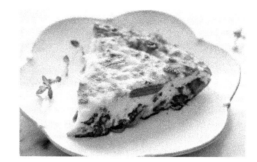

SERVING
4 People

Ingredients

- 4 Bacon slices, chopped
- Salt and black pepper
- 8 eggs, whisked
- 1 bunch Asparagus, trimmed and chopped

Steps to Cook

1. Heat a pan, add bacon, stir and cook for five minutes.
2. Add asparagus, salt, and pepper, stir, and cook for an additional 5 minutes.
3. Add the chilled eggs, spread them in the pan, allow them to substitute the oven, and bake for 20 minutes at 350° F.
4. Share and divide between plates and serve for breakfast.

Barley and Wild Mushroom

TIME TO PREPARE
10 minutes

COOK TIME
40 minutes

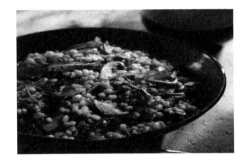

SERVING
3 People

Steps to Cook

- *4 tablespoon oat/soy-based cream alternative*
- *Good grind black pepper*
- *1 onion (140grams), chopped*
- *1 red pepper (160grams), chopped*
- *250grams pearl barley*
- *2 teaspoon olive oil*
- *400gram mixed mushrooms, sliced*
- *2 good pinches of white pepper*
- *1 low-salt vegetable stock*

1. In a large nonstick frying pan, heat the oil, then add the onion and cook for 1 minute.
2. Cook for 2 minutes with the red pepper and garlic, then add the mushrooms and cook for 3 minutes.
3. Set aside a few mushrooms to use as a garnish.
4. Stir in the barley, then add the stock, oregano, and pepper, and combine thoroughly. Bring to a boil, then reduce to low heat, cover, and cook, stirring constantly.
5. Remove the cover after about 25 minutes and continue to simmer for another 10 minutes, or until the liquid has been absorbed and any excess has been boiled off.

- *cube in 700ml boiling water*
- *2 cloves of garlic, crushed*
- *1 heaped teaspoon dried oregano*
- *1 heaped teaspoon chopped fresh basil and more to serve*

6. Cook the barley until it is tender but still firm ('al dente').
7. Stir in the cream substitute and fresh basil, then season to taste with freshly ground black pepper and the reserved basil and mushrooms.

Cabbage Wedges

TIME TO PREPARE
10 minutes

COOK TIME
40 minutes

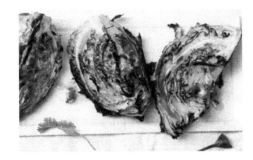

SERVING
6 People

Ingredients

- *1 small head of green cabbage*
- *6 strips of bacon, thick-cut, pastured*
- *1 teaspoon onion powder*
- *½ teaspoon ground black pepper*
- *1 teaspoon garlic powder*
- *¾ teaspoon salt*
- *1/4 teaspoon red chili flakes*
- *1/2 teaspoon fennel seeds*
- *3 tablespoons olive oil*

Steps to Cook

1. Switch on the air fryer, insert fryer basket, grease it with olive oil, then shut with its lid, set the fryer at 350 degrees F, and preheat for 5 minutes.

2. Open the fryer, add bacon strips in it, close with its lid and cook for 10 minutes until nicely golden and crispy, turning the bacon halfway through the frying.

3. Meanwhile, prepare the cabbage, for this, remove the outer leaves of the cabbage, and then cut it into eight wedges, keeping the core intact.

4. Prepare the spice mix and for this, place onion powder in a bowl, add black pepper, garlic powder, salt,

red chili, and fennel and stir until mixed.

5. Drizzle cabbage wedges with oil and then sprinkle with spice mix until well coated.

6. When the air fryer beeps, open its lid, transfer bacon strips to a cutting board and let it rest.

7. Add seasoned cabbage wedges into the fryer basket, close with its lid, then cook for 8 minutes at 400 degrees F, flip the cabbage, spray with oil and continue air frying for 6 minutes until nicely golden and cooked.

8. When done, transfer cabbage wedges to a plate. Chop the bacon, sprinkle it over cabbage and serve.

Family Vegetable Gratin

TIME TO PREPARE
35 minutes

COOK TIME
10 minutes

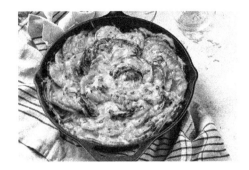

SERVING
4 People

Ingredients

- *1 pound Chinese cabbage, roughly chopped*
- *2 bell peppers, seeded and sliced*
- *1 jalapeno pepper, seeded and sliced*
- *1 onion, thickly sliced*
- *2 garlic cloves, sliced*
- *1/2 stick butter*
- *4 tablespoons all-purpose flour*
- *1 cup milk*
- *1 cup cream cheese*
- *Sea salt and freshly ground black pepper*
- *1/2 teaspoon cayenne pepper*

Steps to Cook

1. Heat a pan of salted water, then bring to a boil. Boil the Chinese cabbage for 2 to 3 minutes. Transfer the Chinese cabbage to cold water to stop the cooking process.
2. Place the Chinese cabbage in a lightly greased casserole dish. Add the peppers, onion, and garlic.
3. Next, melt the butter in a saucepan over moderate heat. Gradually add the flour and cook for 2 minutes to form a paste.
4. Slowly pour in the milk, stirring continuously until a thick sauce forms. Add the cream cheese.
5. Season with salt, black pepper, and cayenne pepper, then add the mixture to the casserole dish.

- *1 cup Monterey Jack cheese, shredded*

6. Top with the shredded Monterey Jack cheese and bake in the preheated Air Fryer at 390 degrees F for 25 minutes. Serve hot.

Vegetarian Zucchini Lasagna

TIME TO PREPARE
10 minutes

COOK TIME
10 minutes

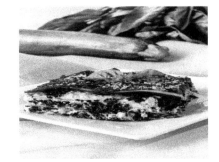

SERVING
6 People

Ingredients

- 1 ¼ pounds zucchini, sliced into lasagna
- ¼ cup chopped fresh spinach
- 1 ½ cup sugar-free and low-sodium marinara sauce
- 2/3 cup mozzarella cheese, shredded
- 1 cup part-skim ricotta cheese
- Fresh basil for garnish

Steps to Cook

1. Preheat the oven to 3750F for five minutes.
2. Place the zucchini slices in a dish and layer with spinach, marinara sauce, mozzarella, and ricotta cheese.
3. Repeat the method until several layers are formed.
4. Top with basil.
5. Place in the oven and bake for 10 minutes.

Bread Sauce

TIME TO PREPARE
10 minutes

COOK TIME
10 minutes

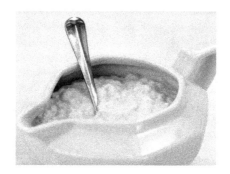

SERVING
2 People

Ingredients

- 125grams fresh
- 8 peppercorns
- 10 grams vegetable oil spread
- Wholemeal breadcrumbs
- 1 medium onion, peeled
- 600ml whole milk
- 10 cloves
- 1 bay leaf

Steps to Cook

1. Using the cloves to pierce the onion, put it in a pan with the milk, bay leaf, and peppercorns.
2. Bring to a low simmer, then remove from the heat and set aside for 2 hours to let the flavors evolve.

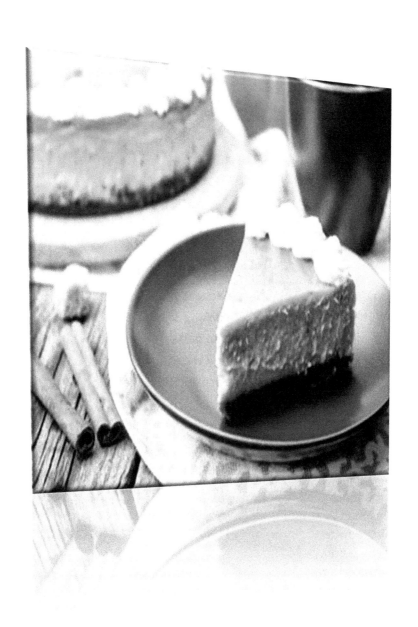

Dessert Recipes

Chocolate Banana Cake

TIME TO PREPARE
10 minutes

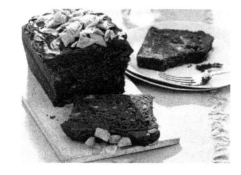

COOK TIME
30 minutes

SERVING
12 People

Ingredients

- *1 cup ripe bananas, mashed*
- *1-1/3 cups all-purpose flour*
- *3 tablespoons cocoa, crushed*
- *1 cup low-fat milk*
- *2 teaspoons vanilla extract*
- *½ teaspoon baking soda*
- *1 teaspoon baking powder*
- *1/3 cup butter*
- *½ teaspoon salt*
- *½ cup of water*
- *Cooking spray*

Steps to Cook

1. Preheat your oven to 350 ºF. Apply cooking spray to your baking pan. Add butter until it is fluffy and light.
2. Add the eggs and vanilla. Beat after each addition. Now stir the water in.
3. Whisk together the milk, flour, baking powder, cocoa, salt, and baking soda. Add this to the creamed mix. Combine well.
4. Stir the bananas in.
5. Place in your pan and bake.

Cinnamon Pears

TIME TO PREPARE
10 minutes

COOK TIME
7 minutes

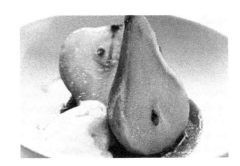

SERVING
4 People

Ingredients

- *4 firm pears, peel*
- *1/2 tsp. nutmeg*
- *1/3 cup sugar*
- *1 tsp. ginger*
- *1 1/2 tsp. cinnamon*
- *1 cinnamon stick*
- *1 cup of orange juice*

Steps to Cook

1. Add orange juice and all spices into the instant pot. Place trivet into the pot.
2. Arrange pears on top of the trivet.
3. Closure pot with lid and cook on manual high pressure for 7 minutes. Once done, allow to release pressure naturally then open the lid. Carefully remove pears from the pot and set them aside.
4. Discard cinnamon stick and cloves from the pot. Add sugar to the pot and set the pot on sauté mode. Cook sauce until thickened.
5. Pour sauce over pears and serve.

Fueling Mousse

TIME TO PREPARE
5 minutes

COOK TIME
3 minutes

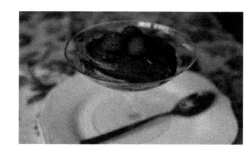

SERVING
2 People

Ingredients

- *1 packet of hot cocoa*
- *½ cup sugar-free gelatin*
- *1 tablespoon light cream cheese*
- *2 tablespoons cold water*
- *¼ cup crushed ice*

Steps to Cook

1. Place all ingredients in a blender. Pulse until smooth.
2. Pour into glass and place in the fridge to set.
3. Serve chilled.

Blueberry Cupcakes

TIME TO PREPARE
10 minutes

COOK TIME
25 minutes

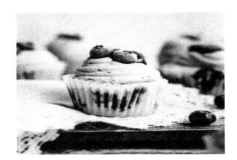

SERVING
6 People

Ingredients

- *2 eggs, lightly beaten*
- *1/4 cup butter, softened*
- *1/2 tsp. baking soda*
- *1 tsp. baking powder*
- *1 tsp. vanilla extract*
- *1/2 fresh lemon juice*
- *1 lemon zest*
- *1/4 cup sour cream*
- *1/4 cup milk*
- *1 cup of sugar*
- *3/4 cup fresh blueberries*
- *1 cup all-purpose flour*
- *1/4 tsp. salt*

Steps to Cook

1. Swell all ingredients into the large bowl and mix well.

2. Empty 1 cup water into the instant pot then place trivet into the pot.

3. Pour batter into the silicone cupcake mound and place on top of the trivet. Seal pot with lid and cook manual high pressure for 25 minutes.

4. Once done, release pressure naturally, then open the lid. Serve and enjoy.

Maple Cinnamon Meringues

TIME TO PREPARE
15 minutes

COOK TIME
2 hours 10 minutes

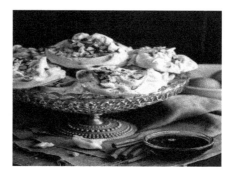

SERVING
6 People

Ingredients

- 4 large egg whites
- 1 cup/240ml maple syrup
- 1/4 teaspoon cream of tartar
- 1/4 teaspoon sea salt
- 1 teaspoon cinnamon plus more for dusting
- 1/2 cup/56 grams almonds, toasted and coarsely chopped
- Sea salt for sprinkling

Steps to Cook

1. Preheat oven to 200 degrees.
2. In a bowl add egg whites, cream of tartar, maple syrup, salt, and set on a pot of simmering water.
3. Remove bowl from heat and whisk to form the glossy peaks. You should whisk for 5 to 8 minutes.
4. Now add the cinnamon powder
5. Drop the meringue mixture on a baking tray
6. Bake for 1 to 2 hours till the meringues are dry
7. Remove from oven, let it cool.

Pineapple Nice Cream

TIME TO PREPARE
10 minutes

COOK TIME
30 minutes

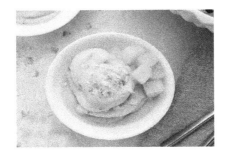

SERVING
6 People

Ingredients

- 1 16-oz. package frozen pineapple chunks
- 1 cup frozen mango chunks or 1 large mango, peeled, seeded, and chopped
- 1 tbsp. lemon juice or lime juice

Steps to Cook

1. In a food processor, process the mango, lemon or lime juice, and pineapple until creamy and smooth. You can add 1/4 cup of water if the mango is frozen.
2. Serve it immediately if you want to have the best texture.

Mini Choco Cake

TIME TO PREPARE
10 minutes

COOK TIME
9 minutes

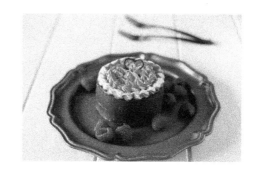

SERVING
2 People

Ingredients

- 2 eggs
- 2 Tbsp swerve
- 1/4 cup cocoa powder
- 1/2 tsp. vanilla
- 1/2 tsp. baking powder
- 2 Tbsp heavy cream

Steps to Cook

1. In a container, blend all dry ingredients until combined.
2. Swell all wet ingredients to the dry mixture and whisk until smooth. Spray two ramekins with cooking spray.
3. Empty 1 cup water into the instant pot then place trivet to the pot. Pour batter into the ramekins and place ramekins on top of the trivet. Closure pot with lid and cook on manual high pressure for 9 minutes.
4. Once done, then release pressure using the quick-release method then open the lid.
5. Carefully remove ramekins from the pot and let it cool. Serve and enjoy.

Cookie Dough Fudge

TIME TO PREPARE
10 minutes

COOK TIME
0 minutes

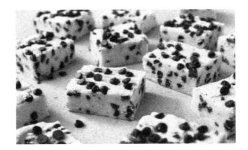

SERVING
4 People

Ingredients

- Cooking spray
- 1/2 c. butter softened
- 3/4 c. granulated sugar
- 1 tsp. pure vanilla extracts
- 1 c. all-purpose flour
- 1 tsp. kosher salt
- 1 1/4 c. mini chocolate chips, divided
- 14-oz. can sweeten condensed milk
- 1 1/2 c. melted white chocolate

Steps to Cook

1. Grease the pan with cooking spray.
2. Now in a bowl beat butter, sugar, and vanilla to form the smooth mixture.
3. Place flour in a bowl and warm it.
4. Add flour and salt to the butter mixture. Beat it and add 1 cup chocolate chips.
5. In other bowl, mix condensed milk, melted chocolate and add in cookie dough mixture,
6. Pour the mixture into a baking pan, add chocolate chips to the top layer.
7. Refrigerate until fudge is formed. Remove the pan and slice it.

Dark Chocolate Cake

TIME TO PREPARE
10 minutes

COOK TIME
30 minutes

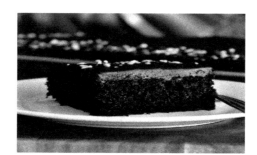

SERVING
10 People

Ingredients

- *1 cup almond flour 3 eggs*
- *2 tablespoons almond flour*
- *1/4 teaspoon salt*
- *1/2 cup Swerve Granular*
- *3/4 teaspoon vanilla extract*
- *2/3 cup almond milk, unsweetened*
- *1/2 cup cocoa powder*
- *6 tablespoons butter, melted*
- *1 1/2 teaspoon baking powder*
- *3 tablespoon unflavored whey protein powder or egg white protein powder*

Steps to Cook

1. Grease the slow cooker well.
2. Whisk the almond flour together with cocoa powder, sweetener, whey protein powder, salt, and baking powder in a bowl. Then stir in butter along with almond milk, eggs, and the vanilla extract until well combined, and then stir in the chocolate chips if desired.
3. When done, pour into the slow cooker. Allow cooking for 2-2 1/2 hours on low.
4. When through, turn off the slow cooker and let the cake cool for about 20-30 minutes.
5. When cooled, cut the cake into pieces and serve warm with lightly sweetened whipped cream. Enjoy

- *1/3 cup sugar-free chocolate chips, optional*

Yogurt Custard

TIME TO PREPARE
10 minutes

COOK TIME
20 minutes

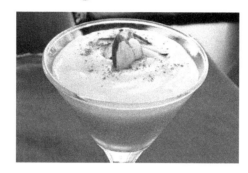

SERVING
6 People

- 1 cup plain yogurt
- 1 1/2 tsp. ground cardamom
- 1 cup sweetened condensed milk
- 1 cup milk

1. Add all ingredients into the heat-safe bowl and stir to combine. Cover bowl with foil.
2. Pour 2 cups of water into the instant pot then place the trivet in the pot, then place the bowl on top of the trivet.
3. Closure pot with lid and cook on manual high pressure for 20 minutes.
4. Once done, release pressure naturally for 20 minutes and then release it using the quick-release method. Open the lid.
5. Once the custard bowl is cool, then place it in the refrigerator for 1 hour. Serve and enjoy.

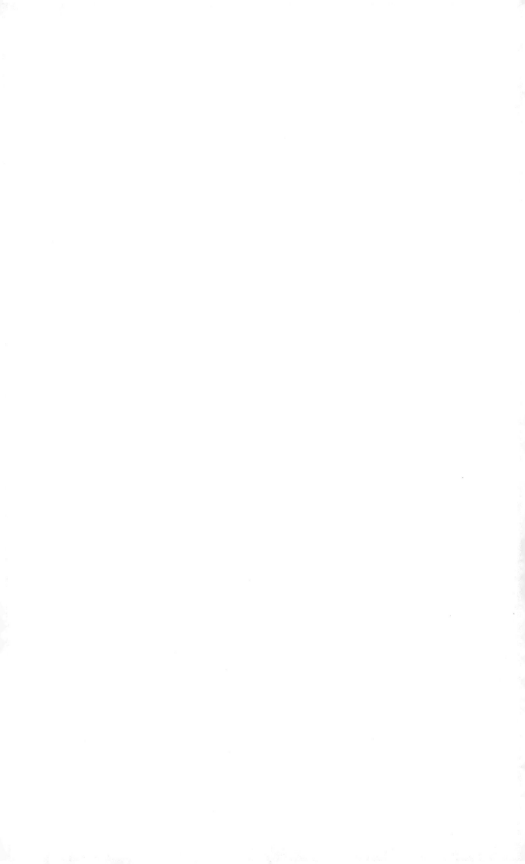

CPSIA information can be obtained
at www.ICGtesting.com
Printed in the USA
BVHW052248070421
604338BV00007B/620